Medical Cell Biology
made memorable

Robert I. Norman BSc PhD

Senior Lecturer in Medical Biochemistry, Department of Medicine, University of Leicester, UK

David Lodwick BSc PhD

Lecturer in Molecular Biology, Department of Medicine, University of Leicester, UK

Illustrated by Robert Britton and Ethan Danielson

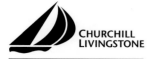
CHURCHILL
LIVINGSTONE

EDINBURGH LONDON NEW YORK PHILADELPHIA SAN FRANCISCO SYDNEY TORONTO 1999

CHURCHILL LIVINGSTONE
A Division of Harcourt Brace and Company Limited

© Churchill Livingstone, a division of Harcourt Brace and Company Limited 1999

◗ is a registered trademark of Harcourt Brace and Company Limited

First Edition 1999

ISBN 0443 05815 6

British Library of Cataloguing in Publication Data
A catalogue record for this book is available from the British Library.

Library of Congress Cataloging in Publication Data
A catalog record for this book is available from the Library of Congress.

Medical knowledge is constantly changing. As new information becomes available, changes in treatment, procedures, equipment and the use of drugs become necessary. The authors and the publisher have, as far as it is possible, taken care to ensure that the information given in this text is accurate and up to date. However, readers are strongly advised to confirm that the information, especially with regard to drug usage, complies with current legislation and standards of practice.

Publisher: Michael Parkinson
Project editor: Jim Killgore
Designer: Sarah Cape
Project controller: Nancy Arnott

The
publisher's
policy is to use
**paper manufactured
from sustainable forests**

Printed in China
EPC/01

Preface

Over recent years medical education has been changing, with much greater emphasis being placed on student-centred learning. Medical students now ask for succinct source materials from which they can quickly gain an overview of a topic; to provide a start point for more detailed reading of relevant material in larger dedicated textbooks and to facilitate their revision for course assessments. This book was designed to provide a condensed synopsis of cell biology to meet the needs of medical undergraduate students and other students studying cell biology for the first time. Our aim was to prepare an affordable book to allow students to develop rapidly a general understanding of areas of cell biology at a level appropriate to first and second year medical studies. A basic understanding of structural biochemistry, the properties of enzymes and metabolic pathways is assumed. Cellular aspects of immunology are not covered by this book as this topic is covered well by another title in this 'series': *Medical Immunology for Students* by J.H.L. Playfair and P.M. Lydyard.

The book is divided into 13 chapters, in a way in which we hope will complement the variety of modular teaching styles in different medical schools. *Cellular organization: organelle structure and function* describes the major membrane bounded structures within the cell and their role in cell biology. Short chapters on *Genes and gene expression* and *Proteins: the molecular basis of cell machinery* are included to help readers unfamiliar with these basic concepts. *Membranes and membrane transport* introduces the properties of biological membranes and considers the specific transport of substances across these barriers. The function of cellular organelles is expanded in *Organelles: compartmentalization of cellular functions and protein targeting*. Three chapters then follow concerning cell signalling. *Cell to cell signalling: chemical signalling and signal transduction* across membranes considers the way chemical messages are recognized by cells and how the information from signal recognition is transduced across the cell membrane. The variety of potential responses within the cell are discussed in *Signal transduction: intracellular signalling pathways*. How cells generate a resting membrane potential and use this in electrical signal propagation within excitable cells is discussed in *Signal transduction: electrical signalling*. The interactions of structural elements of cells that make up cell cytoskeletons and the contractile apparatus of muscle cells are considered in *The cytoskeleton and muscle contraction*. *Adhesion molecules* and *The extracellular matrix* cover the variety of structures that permit specific direct interactions between adjacent cells and the substratum and the co-ordination of cell adhesion and the intracellular control of the cytoskeleton in cell movement is discussed in *Cell migration/motility*. The last chapter, *Cell growth, cell division and the cell cycle* is concerned with the processes underlying the proliferation of cells in tissues and the control of cell numbers by programmed cell death. Consideration is also given to the consequences of dysfunction in these processes in the development of cancer.

This book is a descriptive account of the major processes in cell biology and we have not discussed the considerable scientific findings that underpin our current understanding. However, we have included three appendices that summarize the Tools of molecular biology. Biochemical, immunological and cell biological methods are described in Appendix 1. A summary of Genetic methods is given in Appendix 2 and methods used in electrical recording (electrophysiology) from cells are outlined in Appendix 3.

The material in this book is organized into double-page units consisting of a page of text supported by a facing page of figures to facilitate learning. Topics of direct clinical relevance are highlighted in shaded boxes marked with a syringe icon and related areas of cell biology in different sections of the book are cross-referenced. For the interested reader requiring more detailed coverage, we have included a short list of suggested additional reading at the end of most chapters. Tutorial sections containing revision questions with short answers are included at the end of most chapters to help students assess their understanding of different topics. We hope that students and tutors alike will find this condensed account of medical cell biology a useful learning aid.

Leicester   R.I.N.
1998   D.L.

Acknowledgements

We dedicate this book to our families, to Carole and Michael, and Alison and Anna.

We should like to acknowledge our colleagues in the University of Leicester for their help and advice during the preparation of this text. In particular, we would like to thank Dr. Clive Bagshaw, Dr. Nick Brindle, Dr. John Challiss, Professor David Critchley, Dr. Noel Davies, Dr. Tim Harrison, Dr. Christian Kemp, Dr. Leong Ng, Dr. Raj Patel, Dr. John Quayle, Professor Nick Standen, Dr. Rosemary Walker, Dr. Christine Wells for commenting on early drafts of chapters. For their many comments we are grateful but we take full responsibility for any remaining inaccuracies. We also thank Mrs Evaline Roberts, Dr. Arthur J. Rowe, Professor Carole M. Hackney, Dr. Jim Norman and Dr. Christine Wells for kindly providing micrographs to illustrate the text. Finally, we acknowledge that none of this text would have been possible without the endeavour of cell biologists around the world and we are indebted to the authors of the wide range of material, textbooks, reviews and original papers which we have used in compiling this text.

We gratefully acknowledge permission for the use of the following illustrations:

- Figs 4.5 & 4.8 From Houslay MD, Stanley KK 1984 *Dynamics of Biological Membranes: Influence on Synthesis, Structure and Function*. John Wiley & Sons Limited. Figs. 2.18 and 4.12, respectively.
- Figs 4.9, 4.26, 5.2, 5.9, 9.5, 9.20, 10.4, 10.6, 10.8, 10.12 From Alberts B, Bray D, Lewis J, Raff M, Roberts K, Watson JD 1994 *Molecular Biology of the Cell*, 3rd edn. Garland Publishing, Inc. Figs. 11-1, 11-13, 8-30, 12-23, 12-24, 12-25, 16-14, 16-41, 19-2, 19-7, 19-12, 19-28,
- Figs. 4.15, 9.19, 9.21, 11.2, 12.1, 12.2 From Alberts B, Bray D, Lewis J, Raff M, Roberts K, Watson JD 1983 *Molecular Biology of the Cell*, 1st edn. Garland Publishing, Inc. Figs. 6-48, 10-23, 10-30, 12-53, 10-87, 10-86, respectively.
- Fig. 5.7 From Walter P, Gilmore R, Blobel G 1984 *Cell*:38:5-8 Cell Press.
- Fig. 5.11 With Permission of Professor D Goldberg
- Fig. 5.13 From Nakanishi S, Inoue A, Kitu T, Nakamura M, Chang AC, Cohen SN, Numa S 1979 *Nature* 278:423-427 MacMillan Magazines Ltd. Fig. 4
- Fig. 5.16 From Rothman JE 1994 *Nature* 372:55-63 MacMillan Magazines Ltd. Fig. 4
- Figs. 6.2 & 6.3 From Hardie DG 1991 *Biochemical Messengers: Hormones, Neurotransmitters and Growth Factors*. Chapman & Hall Figs. 2.1 & 2.2
- Fig. 6.5 From Yarden Y, Escobedo JA, Kuang W-K, Yang-Feng TL, Daniel TO et. al. 1986 *Nature* 372:226-232 MacMillan Magazines Ltd. Fig. 6
- Table 7.3 From Cooper DMF, Mons N, Karpen JW. 1995 *Nature* 374:421-424 MacMillan Magazines Ltd. Table 1
- Fig. 8.8 From Rettig J, Heinemann SH, Wunder F, Lorra C, Parcej DN, Dolly JO, Pongs O 1994 *Nature* 369:289-294 MacMillan Magazines Ltd. Fig. 2
- Fig. 10.7 From Campbell KP 1995 *Cell* 80:675-679 Cell Press Fig. 1
- Fig. 11.4 From Colognato-Pyke H, O'Rear JJ, Yamada Y, Carbonetto S, Yi-Shan Cheng, Yurchenco P 1995 *The Journal of Biological Chemistry* 270:9398-9406 American Society for Biochemisty and Molecular Biology, Inc. Fig. 1
- Figs. 11.5 & 11.6 Iozzo RV & Murdoch AD 1996 *The FASEB Journal* 10:598-614 Figs 1 & 3, respectively
- Fig. 12.3 From Harris AK 1994 *International Review of Cytology* 80:35-68 Academic Press Limited Fig. 4
- Fig. 13.2 From Grana X & Premkumar Reddy E 1995 *Oncogene* 11:211-219 Stockton Press Fig. 1
- Fig. 13.6 With permission Professor A Kornberg
- Fig. 13.15 From Kinzler KW & Vogelstein B 1996 *Cell* 87:159-170 Cell Press Fig. 7

Contents

Appendices

Cellular organization: organelle structure and function

The cell (Fig. 1.1) is the smallest functional unit of living organisms and tissues. Cellular contents are delineated by a selectively permeable plasma membrane, which permits control over the internal environment. Cells are classified as **prokaryotic** or **eukaryotic** on the basis of the absence or presence of a nucleus, respectively. Viruses are non-cellular life-forms (Fig. 1.1A) that are dependent on a suitable host cell for their replication.

Prokaryotic cells, represented by bacteria (Fig. 1.1B), are relatively small (1–5 μm diameter) simple cells that are essentially devoid of discrete intracellular membrane structures. All of the cellular contents, including the single circular genomic DNA molecule, are contained within the cytoplasm. Often prokaryotic cells are surrounded by a protective crosslinked lattice that forms a cell wall.

Eukaryotic cells (Fig. 1.1C) of higher organisms, including humans, are larger than prokaryotic cells, ranging between 10 and 100 μm in length. In addition to the packaging of multiple linear strands of DNA in the membrane-bounded nucleus, eukaryotic cells contain other membrane-bounded structures, termed **organelles**, which compartmentalize cellular functions and permit greater cellular specialization and diversity. Even in the cytosol or cytoplasm there is a degree of molecular compartmentalization. A complex crosslinked network of structural proteins that extends from specialized contacts in the plasma membrane, involved in cell–cell and cell–substratum interactions, to dense structures surrounding the cell nucleus forms an intracellular **cytoskeleton**. This acts to maintain the basic cell shape and also has important dynamic functions where it contributes to cellular processes such as the movement of organelles, endocytosis, secretion and cell division. The cytoskeleton also microcompartmentalizes the cytoplasm by restricting free Brownian diffusion and may help to localize individual enzymes catalysing sequential reactions into the same cell regions such that metabolites may be channelled from one enzyme to the next, increasing the efficiency of the pathway overall.

The **cytosol** or **cytoplasm** is the largest compartment in eukaryotic cells and constitutes about half the cell volume. It contains water and dissolved ions, metabolites, building blocks, proteins and ribonucleic acids and is the location of many metabolic pathways.

Organelles with double membranes

The nucleus

With the exception of mature red blood cells, every eukaryotic cell contains a **nucleus** (8 μm diameter) (see Fig. 5.1). The **nuclear matrix** or **nucleoplasm** of each nucleus contains a complete copy of the genomic DNA, which is packaged with protein into **chromosomes**, and several regions of **nucleoprotein** (RNA plus protein) called **nucleoli** in which new protein-synthesizing structures, **ribosomes**, are assembled. The contents of the nucleus are surrounded by a **nuclear envelope**, which consists of a double layer of inner and outer nuclear membranes separated by the **periplasmic space**. The outer nuclear membrane forms a continuum with the rough endoplasmic reticulum (ER) and the periplasm a continuum with the ER lumen. Punctuating the nuclear envelope are nuclear pores (7 nm diameter). These complex structures allow the two-way passage of small molecules or proteins but also provide the exit route for newly formed ribosomes and a selective mechanism for the import of larger proteins (> 90 kDa) bearing appropriate nuclear targeting signal motifs.

Mitochondria

Mitochondria are central to cellular respiration and the production of the cellular energy currency, **adenosine triphosphate (ATP)** (see Figs 5.4 and 5.5). They contain the sites of oxidative phosphorylation and enzymes of the citric acid cycle and fatty acid β-oxidation pathways. Mitochondria are, therefore, more prevalent in active tissues and are often localized within cells at sites of cellular activity. These ellipsoid organelles (2–3 μm × 0.5–1 μm) are coated by a smooth **outer membrane**. The **inner membrane**, in which the respiratory apparatus is located, is highly convoluted into **cristae**, which protrude into the mitochondrial matrix. Mitochondria probably originated as bacterial cells which entered a symbiotic relationship with eukaryotic cells. As such, vestigial DNA genome molecules are still found in mitochondria encoding a limited number of mitochondrial components. Most of the mitochondrial proteins are encoded by the nuclear genome and are transported into the mitochondrion after synthesis in the cell cytosol.

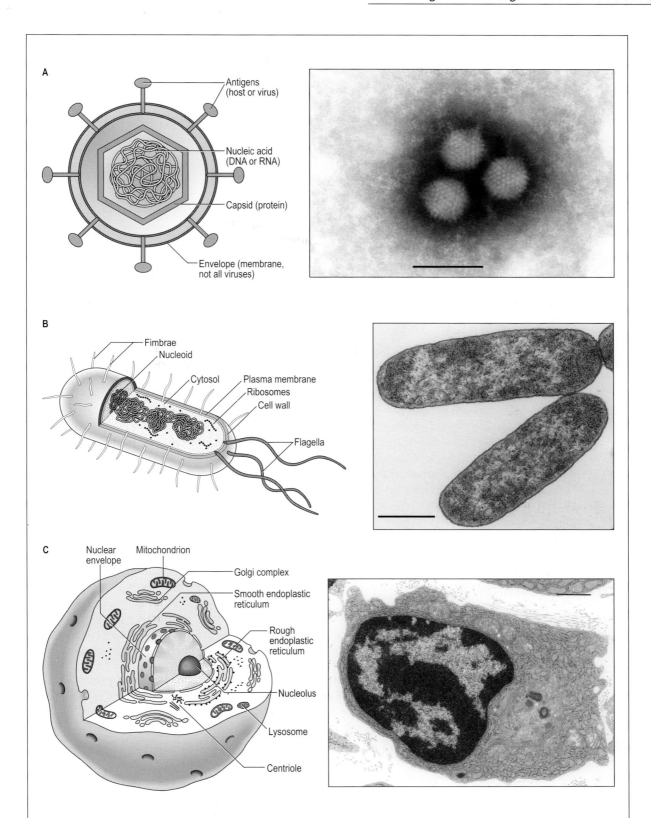

Fig. 1.1 Structure of prokaryotic and eukaryotic cells. (**A**) Viruses are very simple prokaryotic life-forms and are obligate parasites, i.e. they are incapable of replicating without the assistance of a host cell. Viruses have a simple structure with a DNA or RNA genome enclosed in a protein shell (made up of self-assembling capsid proteins). Some viruses also have an envelope of membrane which they acquire when leaving the host cell by budding. *Inset*: electron micrograph of an adenovirus. Bar = 100 nm. (**B**) Bacteria are simple cells that contain some sub-cellular structures but do not contain membrane-bounded organelles. *Inset*: electron micrograph of a rod-shaped bacteria (*Escherichia coli*). Bar = 500 nm. (**C**) In eukaryotic cells, the nuclear material is contained within an envelope of nuclear membrane and some other cell functions are compartmentalized into membrane-bounded organelles. *Inset*: electron micrograph of a typical eukaryotic cell. Bar = 1 micron. (EMs courtesy of Mrs Evaline Roberts and Dr Arthur J. Rowe)

Organelles with single membranes

Endo(sarco)plasmic reticulum

The **ER**, or **sarcoplasmic reticulum (SR)** in muscle cells, is composed of flattened sacs and tubules (**cisternae**) of membrane within the cytoplasm. These structures often form concentric layers around the nucleus. By electron microscopy, two types of ER are distinguished: **rough ER** and **smooth ER**. Rough ER is covered with ribosomes that are involved in the synthesis of secretory, lysosomal and membrane proteins. Both rough and smooth ER are involved in lipid biosynthesis, detoxification and the delivery of newly synthesized secretory or membrane proteins to the Golgi apparatus. Regions of the ER also form intracellular membrane-bound stores of Ca^{2+}.

The Golgi apparatus

The **Golgi apparatus** or **complex** consists of stacks of flattened smooth membrane sacs and vesicles. A prominent function of this organelle is the post-translational modification of secretory and membrane proteins by sequential glycosylation reactions. The Golgi complex is organized functionally into **cis-**, **median-** and **trans-Golgi** such that distinct modifications are made in each region as a newly synthesized protein moves from the ER through the cis- (close to the ER) to trans-Golgi (close to the periphery of the cell). The sorting of newly synthesized membrane proteins to their cellular destination occurs in the trans-Golgi network, which is associated with the trans-Golgi.

Lysosomes and peroxisomes

Lysosomes (0.5–1 µm diameter) contain hydrolytic enzymes for the breakdown of carbohydrate, lipids and proteins. Sequestration of these activities in a distinct compartment protects cellular components in other regions from breakdown. **Primary lysosomes** are formed by budding-off from the Golgi complex. Fusion with intracellular vesicles (**endosomes**) containing materials taken up by **phagocytosis** to form **secondary lysosomes** is important for the breakdown of materials entering the cell by phagocytosis and fluid-phase and receptor-mediated **endocytosis**. Lysosomes also contribute to the turnover of cellular components (autophagocytosis).

Of similar appearance to lysosomes are **peroxisomes**. These organelles contain enzymes that function in oxidative reactions involving molecular oxygen, resulting in the production of hydrogen peroxide (H_2O_2) and organic peroxides. The compartmentalization of these reactions in peroxisomes protects the rest of the cell from oxidative damage. **Catalase** is an abundant peroxisomal enzyme (up to 40% of peroxisomal protein) whose function is to convert toxic H_2O_2 to oxygen and water.

Complex macromolecular structures

Ribosomes

Translation of the genetic message carried by messenger ribonucleic acid (mRNA) into protein is carried out on large ribonuclear (RNA and protein) macromolecular complexes called ribosomes.

Genes and gene expression

Genes

The genetic blueprint for the cell is carried by **deoxyribonucleic acid** (DNA). DNA is a polymer of just four repeating chemicals called **nucleotides**. The four nucleotides are each composed of unique nitrogen bases (**adenine**, **cytosine**, **guanine** and **thymine**, Fig. 2.1A) and common triphosphate and deoxyribose sugar moieties. The sugar and phosphate groups can become linked to one another by phosphodiester bonds (Fig. 2.1B) to form a DNA molecule. It is the order in which the nucleotides are incorporated into the DNA chain that carries the information. Despite having only four 'letters', this genetic 'alphabet' is sufficient to describe all the 'recipes' necessary to make and maintain a complex organism with thousands of different proteins.

Chromosomes are made from two strands of DNA, intertwined to produce a double helix. This structure, in which two molecules of DNA are arranged head to toe, is stabilized by hydrogen bonding between their respective bases. Adenine (A) pairs specifically with thymine (T) and guanine (G) with cytosine (C) (and vice versa, Fig. 2.1A). This specific base-pairing means that the two strands of DNA are **complementary** in base sequence. That is, wherever an A is found in one strand, a T will be found in the other, and, wherever a G is found, a C will be present in the complementary strand (Fig. 2.2).

The two strands of DNA are described as **sense** and **antisense**. The sense strand carries the coding information that describes the final protein, whereas the antisense strand carries the complement of this sequence in the reverse orientation. The information contained in DNA is organized into functional units, called **genes**, each one carrying the instructions for making a single protein. Within each gene are sequences that direct its expression, as well as sequences that describe the structure of the protein product itself (**coding sequence**). The bases that code for protein are read in groups of three, each triplet (called a **codon**) specifying the incorporation of a different amino acid (Table 2.1).

Before the information contained within the sequence of DNA can be turned into protein, it must be copied into **RNA**. RNA is similar in structure to DNA and binds to it readily, but it contains ribose instead of deoxyribose, does not form a double helix, and uses a fifth base uracil (U), instead of thymine. This step, which is called **transcription**, allows genes to be read individually (or in prokaryotes sometimes in small groups). In eukaryotes, transport of mRNA out of the nucleus allows **translation** (protein synthesis) to be carried out in the cytoplasm. The potential to make many RNA copies of a gene also allows the message to be amplified, thus thousands of copies of a protein can be produced rapidly from a single gene. With the exception of retroviruses (see box), the flow of information is always one way: from DNA to RNA and from RNA to protein.

Reversal of the flow of genetic information

Retroviruses. These are a group of viruses, including the major pathogens hepatitis B and human immunodeficiency virus, that carry their genetic information as RNA. Unlike other RNA viruses, their genomes are replicated through DNA intermediates. To achieve this, retroviruses use a unique enzyme called **reverse transcriptase**, which can copy RNA into DNA.

Prions. Spongiform encephalopathies such as scrapie, bovine spongiform encephalopathy (BSE) or Creutzfeldt Jakob disease are characterized by the finding of large quantities of an abnormal protein in the brain and spinal cord. This material, which contains no viral DNA or RNA, is infectious. In order to solve the puzzle of how this infection spreads, it was suggested that the protein might reproduce by somehow directing a nucleic acid copy of itself to be made. This idea was regarded as heretical because it appeared to reverse the accepted view that information always flowed from gene to protein. It is now thought that the protein is an unusual conformational form of an endogenous protein. The infectious agent replicates itself by converting the endogenous protein into the damaging form.

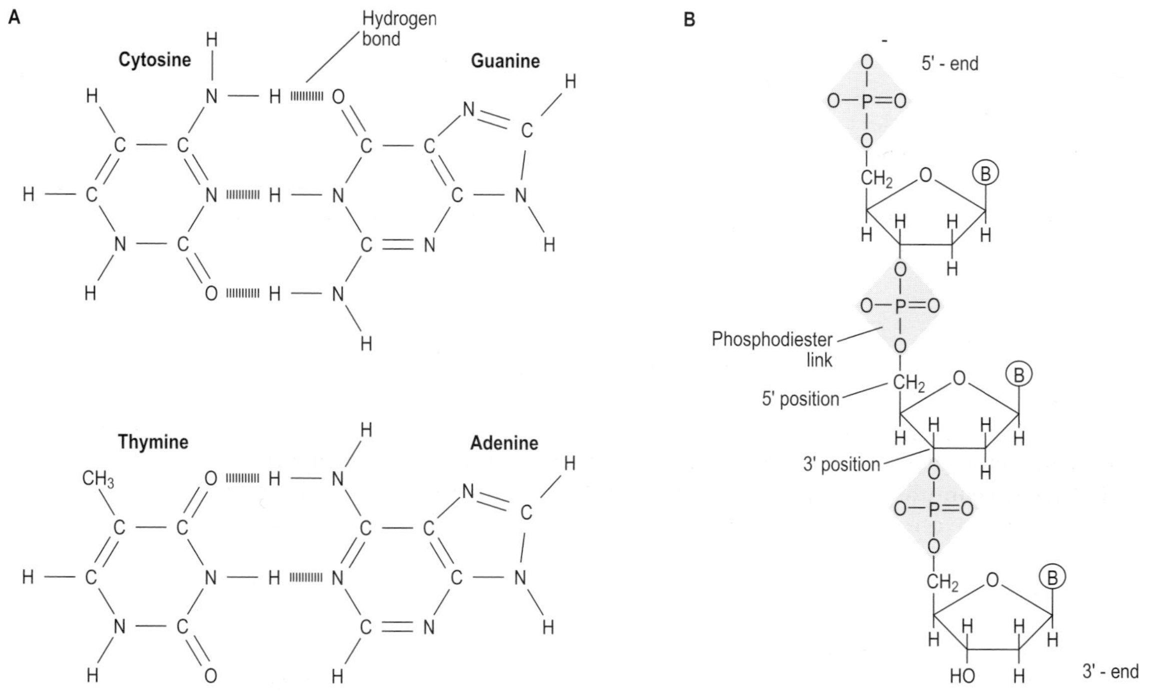

Fig. 2.1 (**A**) The chemical structures of the four bases of DNA and the hydrogen bonding interactions that promote base pairing. Adenine and guanine are purine bases and cytosine and thymine are pyrimidines. (**B**) The backbone of DNA is formed from deoxyribose sugars linked by phosphodiester bonds. B indicates the position of the bases.

First position	Second position: U		C		A		G		Third position
U	UUU	Phe	UCU	Ser	UAU	Tyr	UGU	Cys	U
	UUC		UCC		UAC		UGC		C
	UUA	Leu	UCA		UAA	Stop	UGA	Stop	A
	UUG		UCG		UAG	Stop	UGG	Trp	G
C	CUU	Leu	CCU	Pro	CAU	His	CGU	Arg	U
	CUC		CCC		CAC		CGC		C
	CUA		CCA		CAA	Gln	CGA		A
	CUG		CCG		CAG		CGG		G
A	AUU	Ile	ACU	Thr	AAU	Asn	AGU	Ser	U
	AUC		ACC		AAC		AGC		C
	AUA		ACA		AAA	Lys	AGA	Arg	A
	AUG	Met	ACG		AAG		AGG		G
G	GUU	Val	GCU	Ala	GAU	Asp	GGU	Gly	U
	GUC		GCC		GAC		GGC		C
	GUA		GCA		GAA	Glu	GGA		A
	GUG		GCG		GAG		GGG		G

Table 2.1 The genetic code

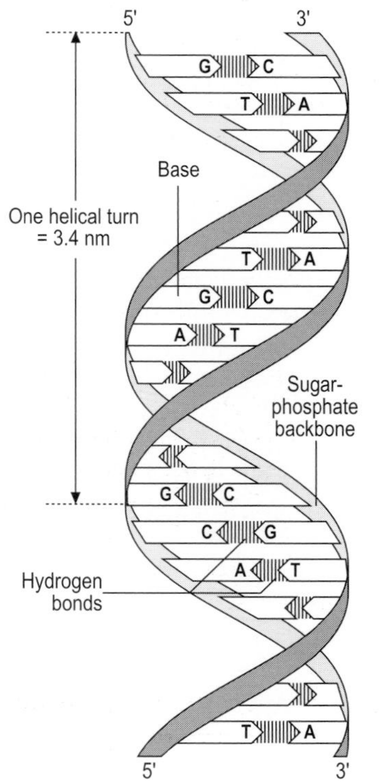

Fig. 2.2 The double helix. Two complementary strands of DNA run antiparallel to each other and are annealed by specific base pairing between A and T, and G and C.

Gene expression

As outlined above, the **genome** contains all the information necessary to replicate an organism. However, proteins, the basic building blocks, are needed in varying amounts, at different times and in different places, each according to their function. Cells must also respond appropriately to external stimuli, such as nutrient availability or signals from other cells. Control of gene expression also explains how a nerve cell and a muscle cell look and act so differently yet share exactly the same set of genes. It appears that this specialization results from differences in expression of relatively few genes. Most genes such as those required for normal metabolic activities (**housekeeping**) are expressed at fairly constant rates in all cells.

Transcription

Genes are transcribed to form primary transcripts by enzymes called **RNA polymerases**, which produce an RNA copy of the sense strand of the DNA by reading the sequence of the antisense strand and synthesizing its complement. Eukaryotes have three different RNA polymerases, each of which transcribes a specific class of gene (e.g. protein-encoding genes are transcribed by RNA polymerase II). Transcription is controlled by the interaction between specific DNA sequence motifs (**cis-elements**) and DNA-binding proteins (**trans-acting factors**). In order to initiate transcription, the polymerase must recognize and bind to sequences called **promoters**, located upstream of the transcription start site. To do this, RNA polymerase must cooperate with other proteins (**transcription factors**) to form an initiation complex (Fig. 2.3), so trancription is controlled by a variety of protein–DNA and protein–protein interactions. Basal transcription is controlled by general transcription factors, but many individual genes may be modulated by the influence of specific **enhancers** or **repressors** binding to cis-elements and affecting the rate at which RNA polymerase initiates transcription. The ability of DNA to bend and form loops means that these trans-acting factors may interact efficiently with RNA polymerase (and each other), even though their binding sites may be a considerable distance apart (cis-elements can be found not only upstream of promoters but also sometimes within the gene itself). Genes that need to be regulated together may share binding sites for particular transcription factors, allowing their transcription to be controlled coordinately by the availability of those factors in the cell. Tissue specificity can work in the same way: if a transcription factor is only expressed in a particular cell type then genes that require it will only be expressed in those same cells.

The 5′-end of the messenger RNA molecule is capped with a methylated guanosine residue (linked by a triphosphate bridge rather than a phosphodiester bond) (Fig. 2.4). This cap is added as soon as the RNA polymerase has transcribed the first part of the message (about 30 bases) and is required both for efficient initiation of translation by the ribosome and for protection of the 5′ end of the growing mRNA from degradation. In eukaryotes the 3′ end of the message is determined by site-specific cleavage rather than simply by termination of transcription. This allows the 3′ end of an mRNA molecule to be varied to produce different protein structures. Once cleavage has occurred, large numbers of adenine residues are added to the end of the transcript to produce a poly-A tail. The poly-A tail protects the mRNA molecule from degradation and acts as a signal for export from the nucleus. Altering the rate at which a gene is transcribed is the most obvious way of controlling the synthesis of its product. However, all the subsequent steps in the path from primary transcript to translated protein, i.e. mRNA processing, export, stability and translation (Fig. 2.5), have the potential to be regulated and many examples exist of genes whose expression is modulated in this way.

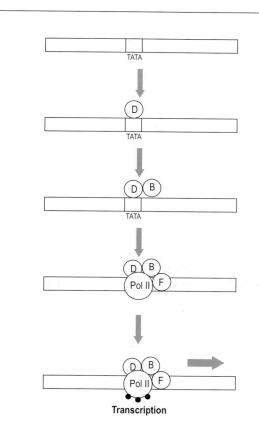

Fig. 2.3 Initiation of transcription. A simplified diagram of the assembly of general transcription factors (D, B and F) and RNA polymerase II (pol II) at a eukaryotic promoter sequence (represented by the TATA box). Both protein–DNA and protein–protein interactions are required. RNA pol II must be phosphorylated (indicated by black circles) before transcription can occur.

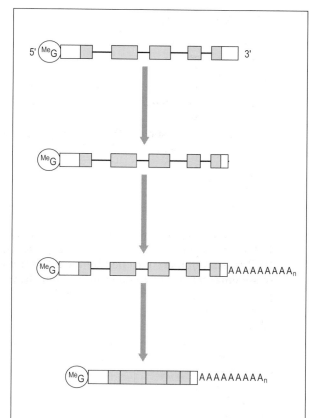

Fig. 2.4 Processing of messenger RNA. (1) The 5′ end of the primary transcript produced by RNA pol II is capped as soon as it is synthesized. (2) The 3′ end of the message is produced by cleavage of the primary transcript. (3) Polyadenylation. (4) Removal of introns by splicing. Coding sequences are shown as filled boxes and untranslated regions as open boxes. Me G, methylated guanosine.

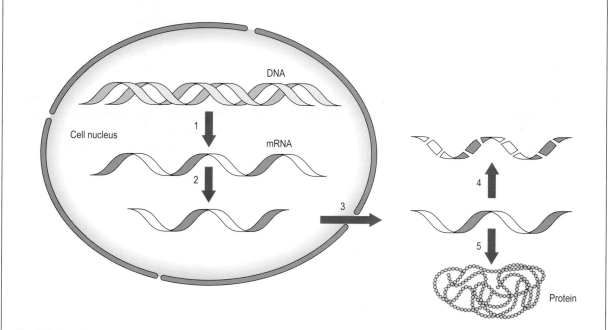

Fig. 2.5 Control of gene expression. The amount of a particular protein that a cell produces can be controlled at many different stages. (1) Transcription; (2) splicing and maturation; (3) transport from the nucleus; (4) mRNA stability; (5) translation.

Splicing of messenger RNA

In prokaryotic organisms, genes are organized as contiguous sequences, i.e. all the code required for making a particular protein is found in an uninterrupted stretch of DNA. In eukaryotes the coding sequence is often interrupted by 'junk' sequences called **introns**, which are transcribed to RNA along with the coding sequences (**exons**) but then removed from the transcript, by a process called **splicing**, to produce a mature mRNA that can then be translated into protein (see Fig. 2.4). Splicing can be used to produce different versions of a protein by choosing whether or not to include particular exons in the mature message (Fig. 2.6). Messenger RNAs remain tethered within the nucleus until they are fully matured. Once all these steps have been carried out the mRNA molecule is ready for export from the nucleus through the nuclear pores into the cytoplasm.

Targeting

Certain proteins need to be specifically localized to the areas of the cell, e.g. mitochondria, where they perform a specialized function. For some this occurs in response to signals carried by the mature protein. For others the information is carried by the amino terminus, so as soon as this part of the message is translated, the growing polypeptide chain, complete with ribosome and mRNA, moves to the correct location (see Chapter 5). mRNAs for a third group of proteins are targeted, without translation, to different parts of the cell by signals carried in their **3'-untranslated regions** (UTRs). Once these messages have been localized, they are translated as normal.

Stability

The rate at which individual mRNA molecules turn over varies between a few minutes and several hours. For genes whose product is required in fairly constant amounts, e.g. housekeeping genes, turnover can be slow with each mRNA molecule being translated many times over a period of hours. Some renewal of the pool of mRNA molecules is necessary to maintain the integrity of the message. Other genes may need to be induced swiftly in response to an external stimulus but then turned off again rapidly once the need for their product has passed. If these mRNAs persist after the stimulus has been removed then so will the response, even though it is no longer necessary, which may be detrimental to the cell. One way to avoid this problem is for these particular mRNA molecules to have a short half-life, i.e. a high turnover. Such mRNAs often have AU rich sequences in their 3'-UTRs, which appear to be a signal for them to be degraded rapidly. mRNA molecules that lack a poly-A tail usually have a high turnover. It has been suggested that the poly-A tail is shortened after each round of translation thus ensuring that older molecules are removed from the pool. An alternative method of control is for certain mRNAs to be protected from degradation by the binding of proteins to specific sequences in their 3'-UTRs.

Translation

The information carried by mRNAs is translated into protein by ribosomes, complexes of **ribosomal RNA** and protein (Fig. 2.7). These assemblies (aided by factors called accessory proteins) identify the **initiation codon** (AUG in eukaryotic and most prokaryotic genes) and make a polypeptide chain by joining the amino acids specified by this and the subsequent codons (Table 2.1). The amino acids are brought to the ribosome bound to specific RNA molecules called **transfer RNAs** (tRNAs). These tRNAs carry a triplet sequence (or **anticodon**) which is complementary to the codon specified by the mRNA. By matching codon and anticodon the ribosome can ensure that it is incorporating the correct amino acid. The codon for the carboxy-terminal amino acid of the protein is followed by one of three **termination codons**, which do not specify the incorporation of an amino acid but rather signal to the ribosome that its job is done.

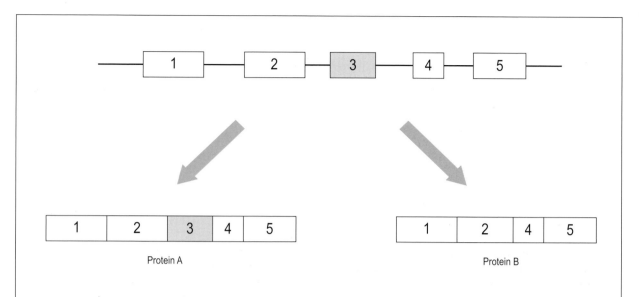

Fig. 2.6 Alternate splicing of mRNA. Two different proteins (A and B) are produced from one primary transcript by inclusion or omission of an exon.

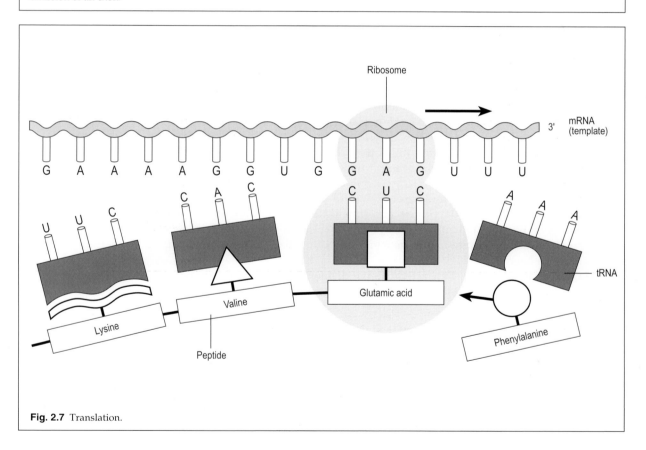

Fig. 2.7 Translation.

Proteins: the molecular basis of cell machinery

Protein molecules define the structural and functional characteristics of cells. The specificity in their structure and function allows them to make highly specific contributions to enzymatic catalysis and the integration of metabolism, mechanical structure and coordinated movements, chemical and electrical signalling, transport and storage, the control of cell differentiation and growth, and in immune recognition.

Protein structure

Proteins are composed of a linear sequence of amino acids (**residues**) linked by **peptide bonds**. Each protein is encoded by a specific gene. The genetic code is transferred from the nucleus to the cytoplasm by **mRNA**, which is **translated** on **ribosomes** into protein sequences. Each codon directs the incorporation of one of 20 possible L-amino acids into the growing polypeptide chain. Amino acids comprise a central α carbon atom linked to an amino and a carboxyl group, a hydrogen atom and, importantly, a variable R group, which defines the character of the amino acid (Fig. 3.1 and Table 3.1). A peptide bond (N–C) is formed when an amino and carboxyl group of two amino acids react (Fig. 3.2). The bond formed is planar owing to its partial double-bond character. This restriction in motion around the axis of the linear sequence of residues, together with steric hindrance between the R groups of adjacent residues, limits the possible structures that can be taken up by the protein. A specific amino acid sequence, therefore, defines a unique three-dimensional structure and proteins are said to be either **fibrous** (elongated structure, e.g. myosin) or **globular** (highly folded structure, e.g. haemoglobin). A genetic **mutation** resulting in the substitution of one amino acid for another residue may produce significant alterations in the protein's structure and, hence, function.

Protein structure can be described at four levels:

- **Primary structure** – the order of amino acids in the linear sequence of the polypeptide chain from the amino (N-) to carboxy (C-) terminus and the position of covalent links between chains, e.g. **-S-S- disulphide bonds**.
- **Secondary structure** – the folding of the primary structure into regular structures, e.g. α-helix (Fig. 3.3A) and β-sheet (Fig. 3.3B), and the stabilization of these structures by **hydrogen bonds** (**H-bonds**).
- **Tertiary structure** – the folding of regions of secondary structure in space to form the three-dimensional shape of the protein and stabilization by ionic and hydrogen bonds, **Van der Waals forces** and disulphide bonds (Fig. 3.4). Tertiary structure also describes the tight interaction of small chemical **prosthetic groups** which contribute to a protein's function, e.g. oxygen binding by haem in haemoglobin.
- **Quaternary structure** – the interaction of distinct polypeptide chains (subunits) to form oligomeric protein complexes and the stabilization of the spatial arrangement by weak bonds or disulphide bonds (Fig. 3.4).

Proteins often can take up more than one thermodynamically stable structure and oscillate between them. Each structure is defined as a **conformation**. When a protein changes shape between two stable structures it is said to undergo a **conformational change**. This may occur spontaneously, on interaction with other chemical entities or in response to electrical events or covalent modification (Table 3.2).

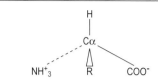

Fig. 3.1 General formula for an L-amino acid at neutral pH.

$$H_3N^+ - C\alpha - COO^- + H_3N^+ - C\alpha - COO^- \rightleftharpoons H_3N^+ - C - C - N - C - COO^- + H_2O$$

Fig. 3.2 The peptide bond is formed between the amino and carboxyl groups of two amino acids with the elimination of water.

R-group properties	Amino acid	R group	Three letter abbreviation	Single letter abbreviation	Specific properties
Non-polar or hydrophobic	Alanine	$-CH_3$	Ala	A	
	Valine	$-CH(CH_3)_2$	Val	V	
	Leucine	$-CH_2CH(CH_3)_2$	Leu	L	
	Isoleucine	$-CH(CH_3)CH_2CH_3$	Ile	I	
	Methionine	$-CH_2CH_2SCH_3$	Met	M	
	Proline	$-CH_2CH_2CH_2-$	Pro	P	Secondary structure breaker
	Phenylalanine	$-CH_2C_6H_5$	Phe	F	Aromatic
	Tryptophan	$-H_2C(CHNH)C_6H_4$	Trp	W	Aromatic
Negatively charged at pH 6–7	Aspartic acid	$-CH_2COO^-$	Asp	D	
	Glutamic acid	$-CH_2 CH_2COO^-$	Glu	E	
Positively charged at pH 6–7	Lysine	$-(CH_2)_4NH_3^+$	Lys	K	
	Arginine	$-(CH_2)_3NHC(NH_2)NH_3^+$	Arg	R	
	Histidine	$-CH_2C(NHCHCNCH)$	His	H	
Uncharged or hydrophilic ('water loving')	Glycine	$-H$	Gly	G	R = H, smallest R group
	Serine	$-CH_2OH$	Ser	S	OH group can be phosphorylated
	Threonine	$-CH(OH)CH_3$	Thr	T	OH group can be phosphorylated
	Tyrosine	$-CH_2C_6H_4OH$	Tyr	Y	OH group can be phosphorylated
	Cysteine	$-CH_2SH$	Cys	C	Forms disulphide bonds
	Asparagine	$-CH_2CONH_2$	Asn	N	Attachment of N-linked carbohydrate
	Glutamine	$-CH_2CH_2CONH_2$	Gln	Q	

Table 3.1 Amino acids found in proteins

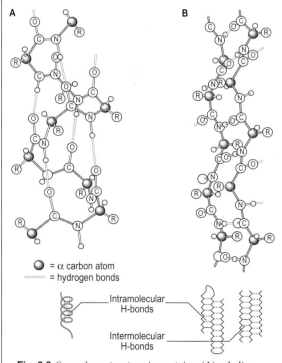

= α carbon atom

= hydrogen bonds

Intramolecular H-bonds

Intermolecular H-bonds

Fig. 3.3 Secondary structure in proteins: (**A**) α-helix, (**B**) β-sheet.

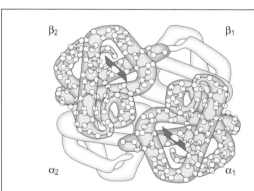

Fig. 3.4 Tertiary and quaternary structure of haemoglobin.

Modification	Description
Glycosylation	Addition of carbohydrate side chains
Hydroxylation	Addition of hydroxyl groups
Mystriolation and palmitylation	Addition of fatty acids
Phosphorylation/ dephosphorylation	Addition/removal of phosphate groups

Table 3.2 Post-translational covalent modification of proteins. Proteins may undergo further covalent modification after synthesis. These modifications may influence the cellular localization of the protein or modulate the final activity of the protein

Bonds in protein

Several bonds are used to stabilize protein structure:

- **Electrostatic or ionic bonds** – formed between charged groups of opposite polarity.
- **Hydrogen bonds** – formed between partial negative and positive charges on atoms arising as a result of non-symmetrical electron distribution around the nucleus. Commonly -O-H. . .N- and -N-H. . .O- (δ^+–δ^-).
- **Van der Waals forces** – non-specific, attractive force between two atoms arising from the non-symmetrical distribution of electrons around the nucleus.
- **Hydrophobic ('water-fearing') interactions** – attractive forces between non-polar groups due to the exclusion of water from the structure.
- **Disulphide bonds** – covalent bond formed from the sulphydryl groups (-SH) of two cysteine residues (R= –CH_2SH) resulting in **cystine**.

Denaturation

Under mild conditions, unfolded proteins can re-fold into their native active structures. However, certain treatments, e.g. high temperature, extreme pH, organic solvents and detergents, induce changes in protein structure from which a return to the native structure is not possible thermodynamically. Such proteins are inactive and are said to be **denatured**.

Protein function

The defined spatial positioning of amino acids in protein structures permits the orientation of R groups to form binding sites, or clefts, for chemical groups. The ability to recognize specifically and interact with other chemical entities is fundamental to the function of all proteins. Proteins can be subdivided on the basis of their functions into structural, binding and catalytic proteins.

- **Structural proteins** may be either elongated fibrous proteins, forming cytoskeletal and contractile structures, or globular proteins, forming adaptors or modulators in structural assemblies.
- Molecular recognition by **binding proteins** allows the interaction with a chemical moiety to be transduced into a cellular event, e.g. receptors for hormones and neurotransmitters, antibodies in immune recognition
- By far the biggest group of proteins are the globular **enzymes** or **catalytic proteins**, which, by binding substrates, provide a microenvironment to accelerate chemical reactions. Enzymes are catalysts and are, therefore, present in the same form at the beginning and end of a reaction. They can catalyse reactions in both the forward and reverse direction (i.e. A + B $\leftrightarrow$ C + D) depending on the concentration of substrates. Note: structural and binding proteins may also be catalytic proteins, e.g. ATP hydrolysis by the contractile protein myosin (see Chapter 9).

Regulation of protein activity

The activity of proteins is often subject to regulation. This may be by:

- direct competition by an inhibitory substance for binding at the active site (competitive inhibition)
- covalent modification of the active site
- proteolytic cleavage, i.e. cleavage of an inactive precursor polypeptide into an active species or termination of an activity by polypeptide cleavage
- binding of a modulator molecule at a second regulatory (**allosteric**) site on the protein to induce a change in conformation and, thereby, function of the protein or
- covalent modification at an allosteric site independent of the active site, which induces a conformational change and affects function.

Allosteric regulation of protein activity by reversible binding of modulators or covalent modification may be inhibitory (non-competitive inhibition) or stimulatory. In particular, **phosphorylation/dephosphorylation** reactions are associated with allosteric regulator proteins.

Membranes and membrane transport

General functions of biological membranes

Compartmentalization

Biological membranes form a continuous sheet-like barrier around cells or intracellular compartments. By restricting the diffusion of most substances between compartments and facilitating the movement of others through a wide variety of protein pores and transport systems, membranes present highly selective permeability barriers that allow the control of the chemical environment in cellular compartments and between the cell and its surroundings.

Communication

Membranes have important roles in biological communication by allowing for the flow of information between compartments in the cell and between cells and their environment. The presence of specific molecules in membranes allows recognition of stimuli in the form of chemical signals (e.g. hormones, local mediators and neurotransmitters), electrical events (changes in membrane potential) and light (retina) as well as secondary signal generation in response to recognition of the primary stimulus, which may be physical, chemical or electrical. Different membranes have specialized functions (Table 4.1).

Membrane composition

Membrane composition varies with cell type but generally membranes contain approximately 40% lipid, 60% protein and 1–10% carbohydrate (dry weight). Note: the membrane is a hydrated structure and hence 20% of the total membrane weight is water, hydrogen-bonded to the hydrophilic surfaces of the membrane.

Membrane lipids are **amphipathic** molecules, i.e. they contain both hydrophilic and hydrophobic moieties.

Phospholipids are the predominant lipids in membranes. They are composed of a glycerol backbone bearing a head group linked through a phosphate group and two fatty acid chains (Fig. 4.1). A range of polar head groups are used (Fig. 4.1) and there is also a great deal of variety in the fatty acid chains. Thus, an enormous variety of phospholipids is found. The presence of a double bond in a fatty acid side chain, which is nearly always in the cis conformation in natural lipids, introduces a kink in the aliphatic chain, which reduces the ability of the phospholipid to pack in a crystalline array and, therefore, contributes to increased membrane fluidity (see below).

Plasmogens are related in shape to phospholipids (Fig. 4.2) but are synthesized via a different route. In addition to the phospholipids, **sphingomyelin** is the only other phosphate-containing membrane lipid (Fig. 4.2). **Glycolipids** are sugar-containing lipids based on the plasmogen structure but with a carbohydrate head group in place of the phosphocholine group found in sphingomyelin (Fig. 4.2).

* **Cerebrosides** are glycolipids with sugar monomer head groups.
* **Gangliosides** are glycolipids with oligosaccharide (sugar multimer) head groups.

Membrane **cholesterol** is found almost entirely in the plasma membrane of mammalian cells where it constitutes about 45% of the total lipid. Four conjugated rings form a rigid, hydrophobic moiety and the hydroxyl group the hydrophilic moiety (see Fig. 4.5).

The distribution of different lipids is tissue specific and related to function.

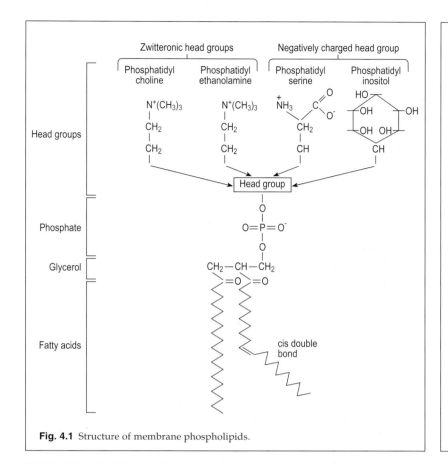

Fig. 4.1 Structure of membrane phospholipids.

Fig. 4.2 Structure of sphingomyelin. Note the similarity to phosphatidylcholine. Attachment of a carbohydrate head group in place of the phosphocholine group results in a glycolipid.

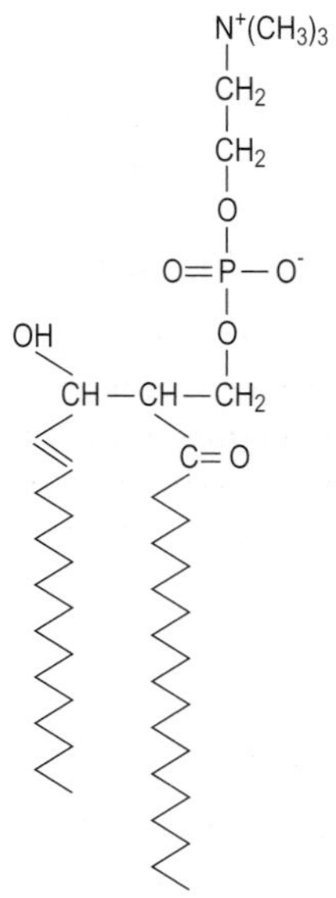

Membrane	Function
Plasma membrane	Separates the cytoplasm from the extracellular environment by forming a continuous barrier around the cell. This limits diffusion of substances into and out of the cytoplasm, protecting the cell from adverse fluctuation in conditions and therefore permitting control of the intracellular environment.
	Punctuated by transport proteins which enable permeability to be regulated.
	Mediates direct communication between cells e.g. contact inhibition, cell adhesion.
	Contains receptor and effector mechanisms for chemical signalling between cells, e.g. hormones, growth factors, local chemical mediators, neurotransmitters
Mitochondrial membrane	Mediates energy conservation by oxidative phosphorylation (c.f. photosynthesis in chloroplasts)
Rough endoplasmic reticulum	Biosynthesis of membrane, secretory and some organellar proteins
Nerve cell – axonal	Conduction of electrical signals
Nerve cell – presynaptic	Release of neurotransmitter
Nerve cell – postsynaptic	Response generation to neurotransmitter

Table 4.1 Some specialized functions of different cellular membranes

Lipid bilayer

Polar head groups of membrane lipids have an affinity for water (hydrophilic) whereas their tails avoid water (hydrophobic). When introduced into water, amphipathic molecules form one of two structures:

- A **micelle**: a spherical structure in which polar head groups face outwards to stabilize the structure by hydrogen bonding with water and the hydrophobic tails are sequestered inside (Fig. 4.3A).
- A **bilayer**: a bimolecular sheet in which hydrophobic tails interact with each other and the head groups face outwards to stabilize the structure by hydrogen bonding with water (Fig. 4.3B). This is the favoured structure for phospholipids and glycolipids in aqueous media. The thickness of a phospholipid bilayer can vary between 5 and 10 nm.

Bilayer formation is spontaneous in water and is driven by the van der Waals attractive forces between hydrophobic tails. The cooperative structure is stabilized by non-covalent forces: electrostatic and hydrogen bonding between hydrophilic moieties and interactions between hydrophilic groups and water.

Model bilayer systems

These include:

- **Liposomes** or lipid vesicles, which are formed when a suspension of phospholipid is exposed to ultrasound (sonication) (Fig. 4.3C). Liposomes have been used for the measurement of efflux of trapped ions and polar molecules. They also fuse with larger membrane systems and may be used to introduce a wide variety of impermeable substances into cells.

Targeted drug delivery

If liposomes could be targeted to specific cells, this method would present a promising means to permit the controlled delivery of drugs to specific cell types. Drug delivery by liposomes is an area of active research interest, e.g. the delivery of cytotoxic drugs to cancer cells.

- **Planar bilayers** can be formed within a hole in a partition between two aqueous compartments (Fig. 4.3d). This system is particularly suited to the study of electrical conduction properties of bilayers.

Both systems have been used to demonstrate that pure lipid bilayers have a very low permeability to ions and most polar molecules.

Dynamics in lipid bilayers

Lipid molecules in a lipid bilayer display four different types of mobility (Fig. 4.4). These motions result in a fluid, two-dimensional bilayer structure in which considerable movement of constituent molecules can occur.

Role of cholesterol in plasma membranes

Cholesterol plays an important role in stabilizing the plasma membrane. The cholesterol hydroxyl group forms a hydrogen bond with the carboxyl group of an adjacent phospholipid (Fig. 4.5). At low temperatures the presence of cholesterol reduces phospholipid packing and, hence, maintains the membrane in a fluid phase, while at high temperatures the rigid cholesterol ring structure held close to the fatty acyl chains reduces intrachain vibrational movements. Thus, cholesterol contributes to relatively constant dynamic properties of the lipid environment in the plasma membrane.

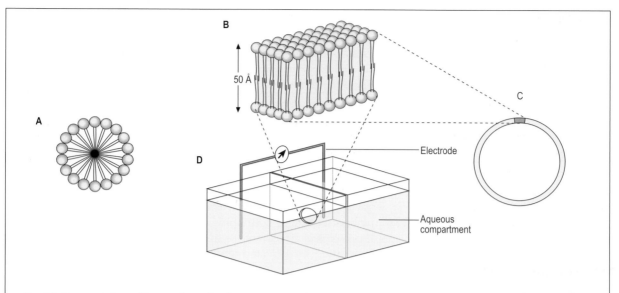

Fig. 4.3 Structures formed by membrane lipids in aqueous media. (**A**) Micelle, (**B**) lipid bilayer, (**C**) liposome, (**D**) planar bilayer.

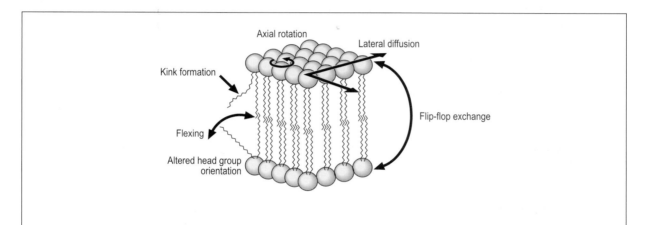

Fig. 4.4 Permitted mobility of lipid molecules in bilayers. (1) Rapid intrachain motion – **kink formation** in the fatty acyl chains, **flexing** of fatty acid chains and phospholipid head groups. (2) Fast **axial rotation**. (3) Fast **lateral diffusion** within the plane of the bilayer. (4) **Flip-flop**: the movement of lipid molecules from one half of the bilayer to the other on a one for one exchange basis. Flip-flop is a relatively rare event, e.g. it may take one day for a phospholipid to traverse the membrane compared with 2.5 μs to migrate the same distance in the plane of the bilayer.

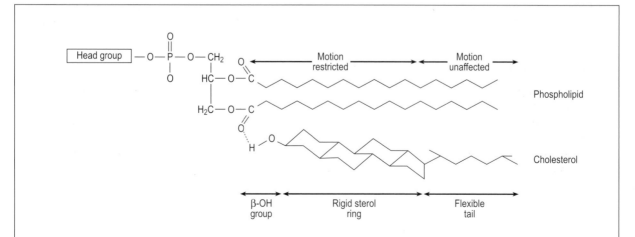

Fig. 4.5 Hydrogen bond interaction of cholesterol with a carboxyl group of an adjacent membrane phospholipid.

Membrane proteins

Membrane proteins (Fig. 4.6) carry out the distinctive specific functions of membranes and include enzymes, transporters, pumps, ion channels, receptors, energy transducers and structural elements. Protein content can vary from approximately 18% in myelin (nerve cell 'insulator') to 75% in the mitochondrion. Normally, membranes contain approximately 60% dry weight of protein.

Lipid mosaic theory of membrane structure (Singer–Nicholson model)

Biological membranes are composed of a lipid bilayer with associated membrane proteins, which may be associated with the surface (**peripheral proteins**) or deeply embedded (**integral proteins**) in the bilayer (Fig. 4.7).

Topography of membrane proteins

There is asymmetry with respect to the distribution of both lipids (Fig. 4.8) and proteins in biological membranes. Directional orientation of proteins is important for function, e.g. a receptor for a hydrophilic hormone must have its recognition site directed towards the extracellular space. Membrane protein topography is generally determined during biosynthesis (see Figs 5.7 and 5.8). It is noteworthy that plasma membrane proteins commonly have complex carbohydrate moieties attached to extracellular domains and are, therefore, **glycoproteins** (see Fig. 5.11).

Mobility of proteins in bilayers

Three modes of motion are permitted for membrane proteins: rotational and lateral movements and conformational changes. There is no protein flip-flop as thermodynamics make this highly unfavourable. Protein movements can be restrained by lipid and protein effects. Integral membrane proteins tend to separate out into the fluid phase or cholesterol-poor regions, and associations with other membrane proteins and/or extramembranous proteins (peripheral proteins), e.g. cytoskeletal proteins, can further restrict movement.

Membranes in disease pathology

The loss of integrity of normal membrane structure is often associated with disease processes. For example, loss of cytoskeletal contacts in red blood cells results directly in the **haemolytic anaemias** (see Chapter 9). **Hypercholesterolaemia** may result from reduced cellular uptake of cholesterol due to mutations in low-density lipoprotein receptors (see later in this chapter). In **diabetes**, important membrane proteins may be destroyed in response to inappropriate protein glycosylation due to hyperglycaemia. Such reductions in insulin receptors and glucose transporters contribute to **insulin resistance** in this condition. Interestingly, insulin receptor and glucose transporter levels are restored on restoration of normoglycaemia in these patients. It is noteworthy also that modification of lipid bilayer fluidity has been associated with a range of diseases such as **diabetes**, **essential hypertension** and **hyperlipidaemia**. However, the relative importance of these changes to the disease processes in these conditions remains to be established.

Action of volatile anaesthetic agents

The anaesthetic potency of the volatile anaesthetics is associated most closely with the lipid solubility of these agents, implicating a hydrophobic site of action and the possibility of a membrane action. The balance of the evidence suggests that this action is not via a modification of lipid dynamic properties and, hence, the functional properties of membrane proteins. A role for membranes in localizing these agents to susceptible neuronal proteins cannot be ruled out.

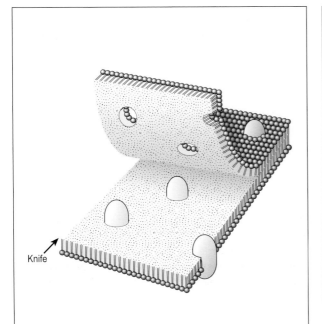

Fig. 4.6 Freeze-fracture electron microscopy provides evidence for membrane proteins. If a fracture of the frozen sample occurs through the middle of the bilayer, surfaces with 'bumps' and 'hollows' are observed under electron microscopy where intramembranous proteins are present or absent in the membrane leaflet, respectively.

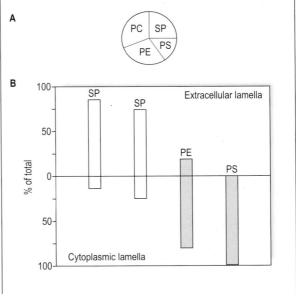

Fig. 4.8 Phospholipid asymmetry in the human erythrocyte membrane. (**A**) Pie chart showing the relative membrane composition of the four major phospholipids. (**B**) Bar graph showing the distribution of phospholipids in the outer and inner lamellae of the membrane. PC, phosphatidylcholine; SP, sphingomyelin; PS, phosphatidylserine; PE, phosphatidylethanolamine.

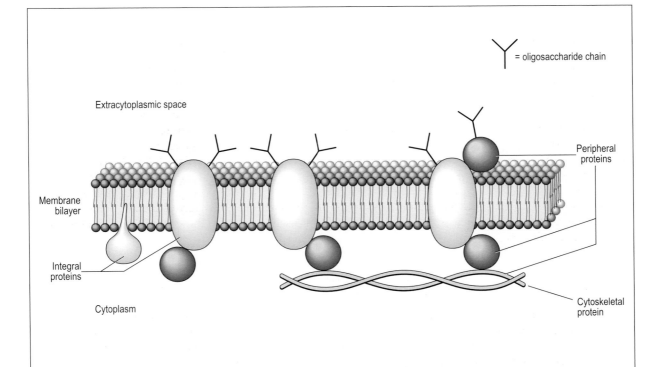

Fig. 4.7 Lipid mosaic model of membrane structure. Peripheral membrane proteins are bound to the surface of membranes by electrostatic and hydrogen bond interactions. These proteins can be removed by changes in pH or ionic strength. Integral membrane proteins interact extensively with the hydrophobic regions of the lipid bilayer. These proteins cannot be removed by manipulation of pH or ionic strength but require agents that compete for the non-polar interactions in the bilayer (detergents, organic solvents).

Membrane transport

Passive transport or diffusion

Non-polar molecules are able to enter and, therefore, diffuse across the hydrophobic domain of lipid bilayers. The rate of **passive** transport increases linearly with increasing concentration gradient.

Movement of water across membranes by osmosis

Permeability coefficients for most ions and hydrophilic molecules in lipid bilayers are very low ($< 10^{-10}$ cm s^{-1}). Surprisingly, membranes are relatively permeable to water (permeability coefficient = 5×10^{-3} cm s^{-1}) and water will diffuse passively across lipid bilayers up the concentration gradient of a solute, the **osmotic gradient**. In some cells, e.g. kidney proximal tubule, the movement of water may be facilitated by specific **water channels**, called **aquaporins**.

Membranes as permeability barriers

The large free energy change that would be required for a small hydrophilic ion or molecule to traverse the hydrophobic core of the lipid bilayer makes the transverse movement of hydrophilic molecules across an intact biological membrane a rare event. Thus, membranes act as permeability barriers to all charged and hydrophilic molecules (Fig. 4.9). The movement of molecules and ions across a membrane is mediated, and regulated, by specific membrane transport systems. Transport processes have important roles including:

- maintenance of intracellular pH
- maintenance of ionic composition
- regulation of cell volume
- concentration of metabolic fuels and building blocks
- extrusion of waste products of metabolism and toxic substances
- generation of ionic gradients necessary for the electrical excitability of nerve and muscle.

Facilitated diffusion

The presence of specific proteins in the bilayer can increase the permeability of a polar substance enormously. For example, the permeability of chloride ions (Cl$^-$) through a phophatidylserine bilayer is very low (permeability coefficient $\sim 10^{-11}$ cm s^{-1}). In the erythrocyte membrane this is increased $\sim 10^7$-fold (permeability coefficient $\sim 10^{-4}$ cm s^{-1}). The protein responsible for the transport of Cl$^-$ is the band 3 protein. This protein does not just form a Cl$^-$ selective pore, but carries out a specific exchange of Cl$^-$ for HCO$_3^-$ (see Fig. 4.22), which is essential to the function of the erythrocyte.

Models for facilitated transport include protein pores, carrier molecules (ping-pong) and protein flip-flop (unlikely thermodynamically) (Fig. 4.10). Facilitated transport is a saturable process as each carrier can interact with only one or a few ions or molecules at any moment and a finite number of transporters are present in the membrane. Thus, as the concentration gradient increases, a maximum rate of transport will be measured when all the transporters are 'busy' (Fig. 4.11). Similar to enzymes, the equilibrium point for the transported species is not altered by facilitated transport.

Some pores are gated, for example:

- ligand-gated ion channels – open or close in response to ligand binding to a receptor site (see Chapter 6)
- voltage-gated ion channels – open and close in response to the potential difference across the membrane (see Chapter 8)
- gap junctions – are closed when the cellular calcium concentration rises above micromolar concentrations or the cell becomes acidified (see Chapter 10).

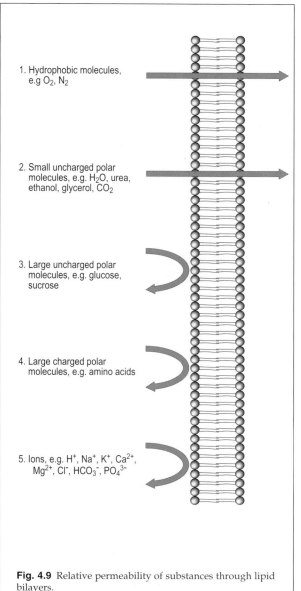

1. Hydrophobic molecules, e.g O_2, N_2

2. Small uncharged polar molecules, e.g. H_2O, urea, ethanol, glycerol, CO_2

3. Large uncharged polar molecules, e.g. glucose, sucrose

4. Large charged polar molecules, e.g. amino acids

5. Ions, e.g. H^+, Na^+, K^+, Ca^{2+}, Mg^{2+}, Cl^-, HCO_3^-, PO_4^{3-}

Fig. 4.9 Relative permeability of substances through lipid bilayers.

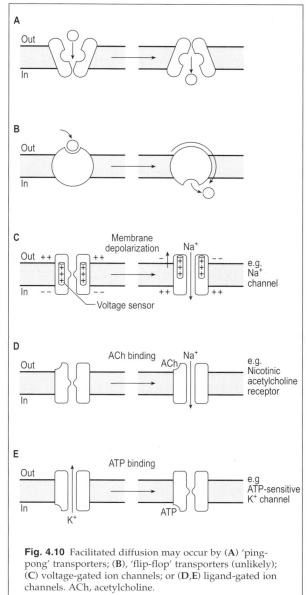

Fig. 4.10 Facilitated diffusion may occur by (**A**) 'ping-pong' transporters; (**B**), 'flip-flop' transporters (unlikely); (**C**) voltage-gated ion channels; or (**D,E**) ligand-gated ion channels. ACh, acetylcholine.

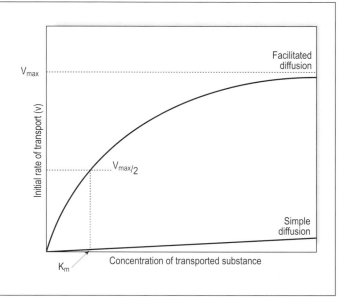

Fig. 4.11 Facilitated diffusion increases the rate of transport of a substance down its concentration gradient and is saturable at high concentrations of the transported substance. Figure drawn assumes a low concentration on the receiving side of the membrane.

Active transport

Whether the transport of an ion or molecule can occur spontaneously (**passive transport**) or requires energy (**active transport**) is determined by the free energy change of the transported species. The free energy change is determined by the concentration gradient for the transported species and by the electrical potential across the membrane bilayer when the transported species is charged (Fig. 4.12).

To overcome unfavourable chemical or electrical gradients, the movement of the transported ion or molecule must be **coupled** to a thermodynamically favourable reaction (Figs 4.13 and 4.14). The free energy to drive active transport comes either directly or indirectly from the hydrolysis of adenosine triphosphate (ATP). For example, the Na^+–K^+-dependent adenosine triphosphatase (ATPase) (Na^+ pump) pumps three Na^+ ions outwards and two K^+ ions inwards, against the respective concentration gradients, at the expense of one ATP molecule hydrolysed (Fig. 4.14). Note: if the pump runs in reverse it can act as an ATP generator. In mitochondria, dissipation of a gradient of H^+ ions is used to drive ATP synthesis via an ATP-dependent proton transporter.

Sometimes the transport of one substance is linked to the concentration gradient of another via a **co-transporter**. This is known as **secondary active transport** because the energy of ATP hydrolysis is used indirectly (Fig. 4.14). Membrane transporters may be driven by gradients of ATP, phosphoenolpyruvate, protons and sodium ions, light and high-potential electrons. Often a sodium gradient across a membrane is used. Examples of co-transport systems include Na^+–H^+ exchange, Na^+–Ca^{2+} exchange and Na^+–glucose co-transport (see below).

Transporter terminology (Fig. 4.15)

When a single solute molecule species is transported from one side of the membrane to the other, the transporter is called a **uniporter**. Other transporters are referred to as **co-transporters**, when the transfer of one solute molecule depends on the simultaneous or sequential transfer of a second solute in the same direction (**symport**) or in the opposite direction (**antiport**).

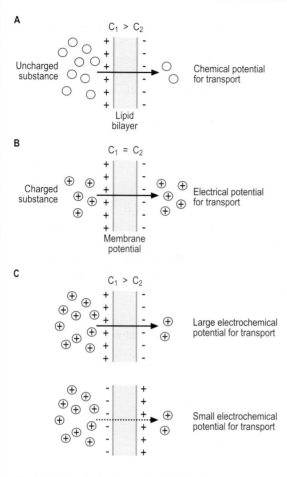

Fig. 4.12 Chemical and electrical driving forces on transported species. c_1 and c_2 are the concentration of transported substance on each side of the membrane.

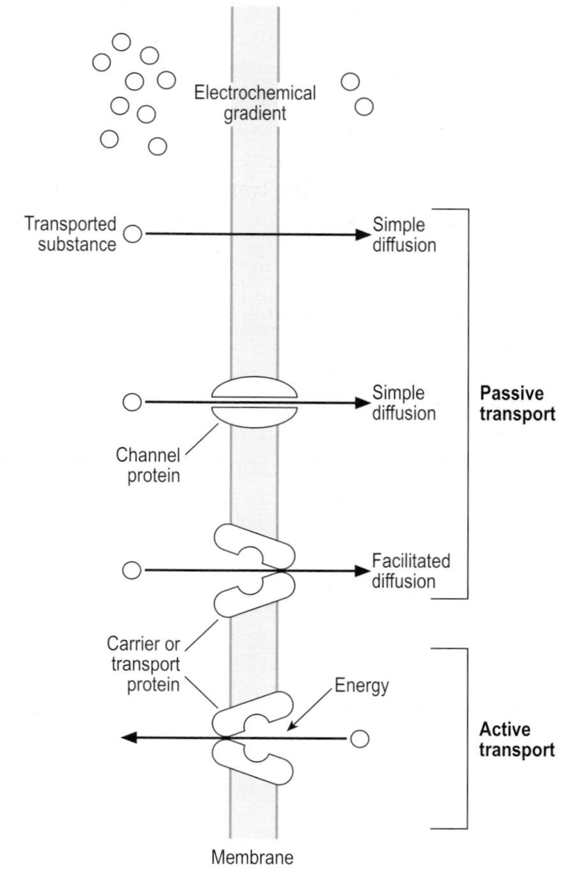

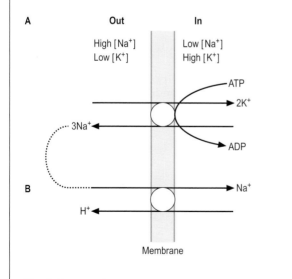

Fig. 4.14 Examples of (**A**) primary and (**B**) secondary active transport. (**A**) Na⁺–K⁺ ATPase uses the energy released on ATP hydrolysis to pump three Na⁺ ions out of the cell in exchange for two K⁺ ions in against their concentration gradients. (**B**) Na⁺–H⁺ exchange uses the Na⁺ gradient maintained by the Na⁺–K⁺ ATPase to drive the efflux of protons.

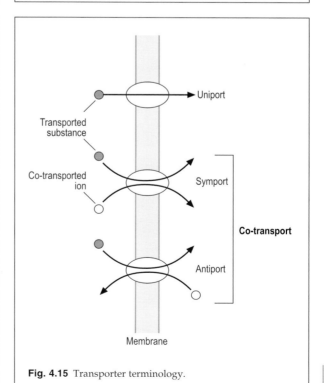

Fig. 4.13 Mechanisms permitting passive and active transport across membranes.

Fig. 4.15 Transporter terminology.

Ion transporters

The movement of ions across membranes is facilitated by specific channel or ion transporter proteins. The opening of channel pores allows the movement of ions down their electrochemical gradient (a combination of electrical and concentration forces on the ion). Transport of ions against their electrochemical gradient requires an active transport process. These can be either coupled directly to the energy of hydrolysis of ATP, known as **ATP-dependent pumps** or **ATPases**, or by secondary active transport processes that use other energy sources.

ATP-dependent pumps

Na⁺–K⁺ ATPase or Na⁺ pump

This plasma membrane transporter is crucial to the maintenance of the gradients for Na^+ and K^+ across the plasma membrane in resting cells (Fig. 4.16). For each ATP hydrolysed, three Na^+ ions are removed from the cell (efflux) and two K^+ ions are brought in (influx). The Na^+–K^+ ATPase is found in all cells and can consume a significant amount of the total ATP produced by a cell. In addition to maintaining Na^+ and K^+ gradients, the Na^+–K^+ ATPase contributes to secondary active transport, the regulation of cell volume and pH and adsorption through epithelia, by sustaining the Na^+ gradient.

> ### Na⁺–K⁺ ATPase inhibitors in the treatment of congestive heart failure
>
> Cardiac glycosides (e.g. digoxin, ouabain), which are inhibitors of the Na^+–K^+ ATPase, are used in the treatment of congestive heart failure to increase the force of contraction (positive inotropy). Increased cellular Na^+ content also reduces the Ca^{2+} extrusion activity of the Na^+–Ca^{2+} exchanger (see below), resulting in cellular retention of Ca^{2+}, which is sequestered into intracellular stores. Release of this additional stored Ca^{2+} on cardiac excitation (see Chapter 7) contributes to the positive inotropism of these agents.

Plasma membrane Ca²⁺–Mg²⁺ ATPase (Ca²⁺ pump, PMCA)

Ca^{2+}–Mg^{2+} ATPases in the plasma membrane (**PMCA**) (Fig. 4.17) present a high-affinity mechanism for the active extrusion of Ca^{2+} against the electrochemical gradient at the expense of ATP hydrolysis to maintain the low $[Ca^{2+}]_i$. In some cells, such as the erythrocyte and myocardial muscle cells, the binding of calmodulin results in a reduction in the K_M for Ca^{2+} and to an increase in maximum activity of the transporter. This response to calmodulin allows cells to react to raised Ca^{2+} levels thereby quickly restoring resting $[Ca^{2+}]_i$. Not all Ca^{2+} ATPases are sensitive to calmodulin. PMCA are also activated by phosphorylation by protein kinases. This is important for the regulation of Ca^{2+} efflux from the cell (see Chapter 7).

Sarcoplasmic reticulum Ca²⁺ ATPase (SERCA)

A second, related, Ca^{2+} ATPase is found in the sarcoplasmic or endoplasmic reticulum (**SERCA**) (Fig. 4.18). This transporter provides for the active transport of Ca^{2+} into vesicular stores in the cell and is an important mechanism in cellular signalling (see page 72). SERCA pumps two Ca^{2+} ions into the sarcoplasmic reticulum for every ATP molecule hydrolysed.

Mitochondrial F₀F₁ ATPase (ATP synthetase)

In addition to using the energy from ATP hydrolysis to drive ion transport across membranes, ion transporters may operate in reverse mode. Most importantly, in mitochondria, the F_0F_1 ATPase, operating in this way, uses the proton gradient established by the electron transport chain to drive the synthesis of ATP from adenosine diphosphate (ADP) and inorganic phosphate (Fig. 4.19).

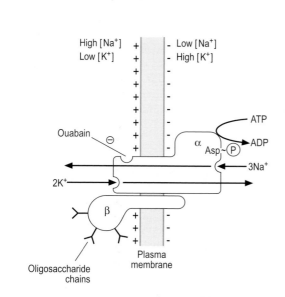

Fig. 4.16 Na⁺–K⁺-ATPase. Three Na⁺ ions are exchanged for two K⁺ ions during each reaction cycle. The Na⁺–K⁺ ATPase is, therefore, **electrogenic**, generating a small outward current and small hyperpolarization of the cell membrane (–5 to –10 mV). Although important in maintaining the ion gradients necessary for the generation of the resting membrane potential (see chapter 8), it is noteworthy that the Na⁺–K⁺ ATPase makes only a small direct contribution to the resting membrane potential. Na⁺–K⁺ ATPase are composed of $\alpha\beta$ dimers or oligomers. The α subunit contains binding sites for Na⁺, K⁺, ATP and ouabain and the catalytic site for ATP hydrolysis, while the β subunit is important for the assembly, maturation and localization of the pump.

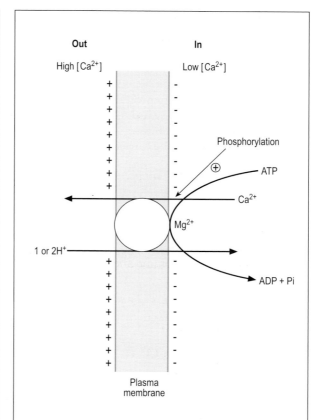

Fig. 4.17 Plasma membrane Ca²⁺-ATPase (PMCA). PMCA require Mg²⁺ as a co-factor and, for every ATP molecule hydrolysed, extrude one Ca²⁺ ion with the exchange of one or two H⁺ ions. PMCA activity is increased in response to phosphorylation by several protein kinases.

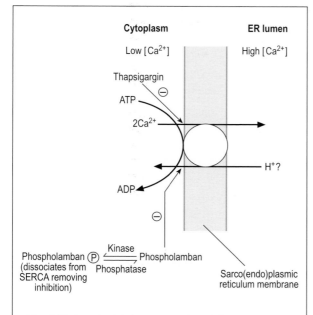

Fig. 4.18 Sarco(endo)plasmic reticulum Ca²⁺ ATPase (SERCA). A regulatory protein, **phospholamban**, binds to and inhibits SERCA in unstimulated cells. Phosphorylation of phospholamban by several protein kinases results in dissociation of the phospholamban molecule from SERCA and activation of the pump. Other inhibitors of SERCA include thapsigargin.

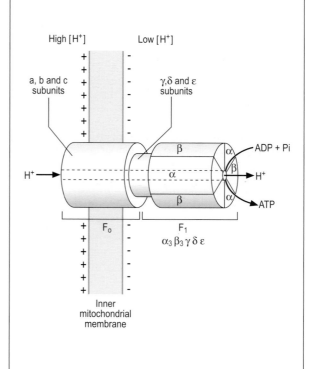

Fig. 4.19 Mitochondrial F_0F_1-ATPase (ATP synthetase).

27

Ion exchangers

Na⁺–Ca²⁺ exchanger (antiport)

Na^+–Ca^{2+} exchange is a high-capacity, low-affinity secondarily active transport system that extrudes Ca^{2+} from the cell by using energy from the influx of Na^+ down its electrochemical gradient and the membrane potential (Fig. 4.20). This plasma membrane transporter comes into operation to pump out Ca^{2+} from the cell after cell stimulation when $[Ca^{2+}]_i$ is raised, e.g. in cardiac muscle. One Ca^{2+} ion is exchanged for the inward movement of three Na^+ ions and, therefore, the transporter is electrogenic. In depolarized membranes the Na^+–Ca^{2+} exchanger activity can reverse and thereby contribute to Ca^{2+} influx, e.g. during the cardiac action potential.

Na⁺–H⁺ exchanger (NHE) (antiport)

This secondarily active exchanger uses the inward electrochemical gradient for Na^+ to expel H^+ from the cell. It is electroneutral, exchanging one Na^+ ion for one H^+ ion across the plasma membrane (Fig. 4.21A). The NHE, which is present in all cells, can function to regulate cell pH and cell volume and is important in cell growth, being activated by phosphorylation in response to growth factors. The NHE can also be activated by calmodulin in response to raised $[Ca^{2+}]_i$. On cell shrinking, influx of Na^+ via the NHE contributes to the restoration of osmotic strength and control of cell volume.

Anion exchangers (Cl⁻–HCO₃⁻ exchangers)

Exchange of anions can be either independent of, or dependent on, the electrochemical gradient for Na^+.

- **Na^+-independent Cl^-–HCO_3^- exchangers** in the plasma membrane mediate the exchange of one Cl^- ion for one HCO_3^- ion and are, therefore, electroneutral. Transport may be in either direction. These transporters can function to load cells with Cl^- ions against the electrochemical gradient for Cl^-, to reduce cell alkalinization by removal of HCO_3^- and to regulate cell volume.

Anion exchange in red blood cells

The best characterized example of a Na^+-independent anion exchanger is the 'band 3' protein of the erythrocyte membrane, which is responsible for the 'Cl^- shift' whereby the movement of HCO_3^- ions into the erythrocyte in pulmonary capillaries and out of the erythrocyte in systemic capillaries contributes to the buffering capacity of the erythrocyte and its ability to transport O_2 and CO_2 in the circulation (Fig. 4.22).

- **Na^+-dependent Cl^-–HCO_3^- exchangers** in the plasma membrane mediate the uptake of HCO_3^- and Na^+ ions with the exchange of Cl^- and H^+ ions, respectively. These transporters are activated by cell acidification and protect the cell from acid load.

Diuretic drugs act on ion transport mechanisms in the kidney

Almost all of the Na^+ that appears in the glomerular filtrate is reabsorbed from the kidney nephron. The driving force for this reabsorbtion is the low intracellular Na^+ concentration that is maintained by Na^+–K^+ ATPase activity in tubular cells. Several transport mechanisms are involved in Na^+ reabsorbtion at different locations in the nephron (Fig. 4.23). Where fluid loss is required to treat oedema and hypertension, block of one or more of the Na^+ reabsorbtion mechanisms with diuretic drugs (Fig. 4.23) can be used to increase Na^+ excretion to produce a hyperosmotic urine and, hence, the excretion of water.

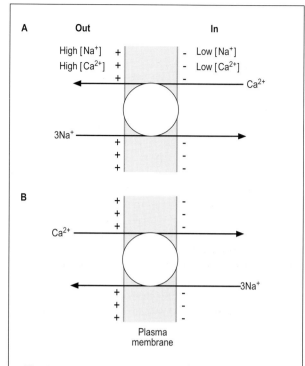

Fig. 4.20 Modes of operation of the plasma membrane Na^+–Ca^{2+} exchanger: (**A**) at resting membrane potential or raised $[Ca^{2+}]_i$; or (**B**) in depolarized membrane or raised $[Na^+]_i$.

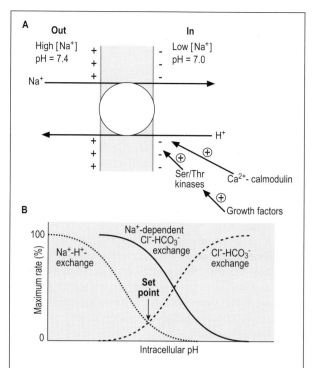

Fig. 4.21 (**A**) Na^+–H^+ exchanger. (**B**) Intracellular pH-dependent activity of Na^+–H^+ exchange, Na^+-dependent Cl^-–HCO_3^- exchange and Cl^-–HCO_3^- exchange. The set point is the optimal intracellular pH.

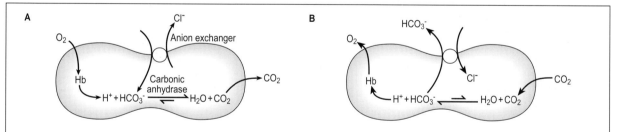

Fig. 4.22 Mode of operation of the erythrocyte anion exchanger (band 3) in (**A**) pulmonary capillaries and (**B**) capillaries in actively metabolizing tissues. Anion exchange is essential to the transport of CO_2 from metabolizing tissues and its release in the lungs.

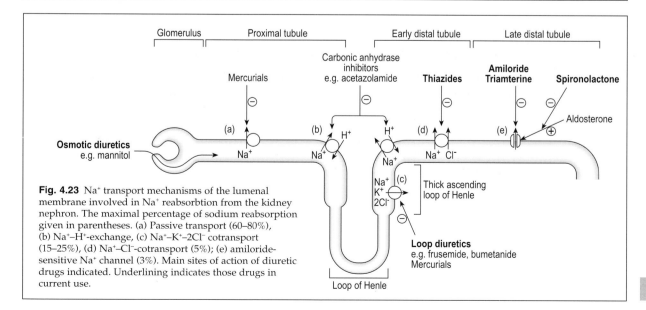

Fig. 4.23 Na^+ transport mechanisms of the lumenal membrane involved in Na^+ reabsorbtion from the kidney nephron. The maximal percentage of sodium reabsorption given in parentheses. (a) Passive transport (60–80%), (b) Na^+–H^+-exchange, (c) Na^+–K^+–2Cl^- cotransport (15–25%), (d) Na^+–Cl^--cotransport (5%); (e) amiloride-sensitive Na^+ channel (3%). Main sites of action of diuretic drugs indicated. Underlining indicates those drugs in current use.

Role of ion transport in cellular physiology

The major roles of ion transporters are to maintain ionic concentration gradients and to regulate cell pH and volume.

pH regulation

When the short-term buffering capacity (PO_4^{3-}, HCO_3^- and protein) of a cell is exceeded, pH is controlled by the transport of H^+ and HCO_3^- ions across the plasma membrane (Fig. 4.24). Most cells possess both NHE and anion exchangers and, additionally, $Na^+-Cl^--HCO_3^--H^+$ counter-transporters and **$Na^+-HCO_3^-$ co-transporters** are present in some cells (Fig. 4.21). Cell acidification leads to activation of acid extrusion by NHE and $Na^+-Cl^--HCO_3^--H^+$ counter-transport, where present. Transporters involved in the response to cell acidification all depend on the electrochemical gradient for Na^+ to provide the driving force (Fig. 4.24). Therefore, the activity of Na^+-K^+ ATPase is crucial to these mechanisms. Cell alkalinization is controlled by the extrusion of HCO_3^- by Na^+-independent anion exchangers.

Volume regulation

Cell volume changes are mediated by the movement of water across the membrane in response to modifications in the osmotic strength of the cytoplasm. Changes in the osmotic strength of the cytoplasm can be achieved by the movement, inwards or outwards, of ionic species or osmotically active compounds, such as sugars. Specifically, operation of the Na^+-K^+ ATPase, by maintaining a low intracellular Na^+ concentration and through the associated movement of other ions, provides the driving force for the passive diffusion of K^+ and Cl^- in response to cell swelling and the $Na^+-K^+-2Cl^-$ co-transport system in reponse to cell shrinking, respectively, and/or the concerted action of proton and anion exchangers (Fig. 4.25). In some cells it appears that swelling operated channels for organic solutes may exist, allowing efflux of small molecular weight solutes to decrease the ionic strength (e.g. myoinositol in the brain, amino acids).

Transport of small molecules

Transporters that mediate facilitated diffusion of small solute molecules, e.g. glucose and amino acids, are often present in cell membranes. Where transport is in the same direction as the concentration gradient for the solute molecule, facilitated diffusion occurs, e.g. glucose uptake into adipose tissue, brain, liver and skeletal muscle (Fig. 4.26). In these tissues, rapid conversion of the glucose entering the cell to glucose-6-phosphate prevents a rise in intracellular glucose concentration to levels that would slow further uptake (Fig. 4.26A). Stimulation of glucose uptake by insulin in tissue such as adipose tissue and skeletal muscle occurs by the recruitment of glucose transporters in vesicles, which are stimulated to fuse with the plasma membrane, thereby increasing the maximum transport capacity of the membrane

Transport of solute molecules may also be active, coupled to the electrochemical gradient for Na^+. For example, glucose transport across intestinal and kidney epithelial cells is driven at the lumenal surface by a Na^+-dependent glucose transporter (Fig. 4.26B). The majority of glucose molecules entering the epithelial cell escape metabolism and pass into the blood down the concentration gradient via facilitated transport through a transport protein in the basal membrane.

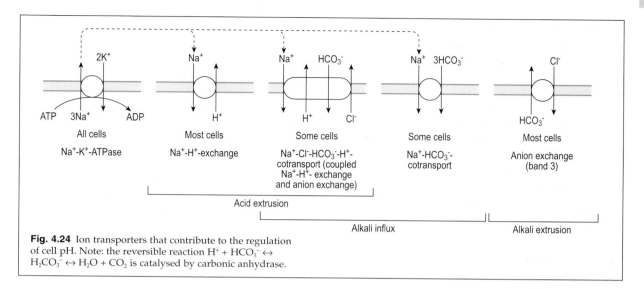

Fig. 4.24 Ion transporters that contribute to the regulation of cell pH. Note: the reversible reaction $H^+ + HCO_3^- \leftrightarrow H_2CO_3^- \leftrightarrow H_2O + CO_2$ is catalysed by carbonic anhydrase.

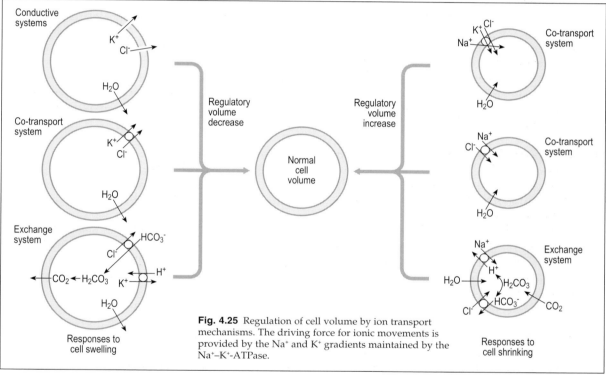

Fig. 4.25 Regulation of cell volume by ion transport mechanisms. The driving force for ionic movements is provided by the Na^+ and K^+ gradients maintained by the Na^+–K^+-ATPase.

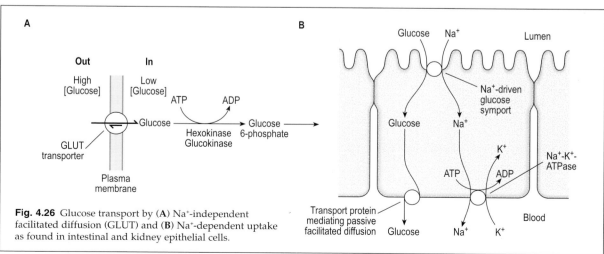

Fig. 4.26 Glucose transport by (**A**) Na^+-independent facilitated diffusion (GLUT) and (**B**) Na^+-dependent uptake as found in intestinal and kidney epithelial cells.

Transport of macromolecules, particles and extracellular fluid

Substances may be taken up into cells by a form of cellular 'ingestion' in which the plasma membrane invaginates and ultimately pinches off to form a membrane vesicle. Such processes are subdivided into **phagocytosis** and **pinocytosis** to distinguish the uptake of particular matter or fluid-phase, respectively.

Phagocytosis

In mammals, phagocytosis is found only in specialized cells, e.g. macrophages and neutrophils. This process permits the clearance of damaged cellular materials and invading organisms for destruction. Uptake depends on binding of the particle to receptors on the plasma membrane. In response to binding, the cell extends pseudopods permitting further receptor interactions and membrane evagination and internalization via a 'membrane-zippering' mechanism (Fig. 4.27). Internalized phagosomes fuse with lysosomes to form phagolysosomes, in which the particulate material is degraded.

Pinocytosis

Pinocytosis is a continuous process, in most cells, leading to the uptake of solutes from the external medium and retrieval of plasma membrane to balance that inserted by the secretory pathways. Pinocytosis occurs by membrane invagination and can be subdivided into two forms: **fluid-phase** and **receptor-mediated endocytosis**. The former permits the uptake of entrapped solutes, while the latter provides a mechanism whereby specific binding to cell surface receptors brings about the selective uptake of molecules into the cell. In most animal cells both forms of pinocytosis occur. Most endocytic vesicles ultimately fuse with primary lysosomes to form secondary lysosomes, in which internalized materials are digested. Most of the internalized membrane constituents, however, are returned to the plasma membrane by, as yet, unknown mechanisms.

Uptake of cholesterol: an example of receptor-mediated endocytosis

Cholesterol is carried in the circulation in large spherical particles that originate in the liver, called **low-density lipoproteins (LDLs)** (Fig. 4.28). Each LDL contains a non-polar core of approximately 1500 cholesterol molecules esterified to long chain fatty acids, surrounded by a lipid layer containing phospholipids, cholesterol and a single protein species, apoprotein B.

Cells that require cholesterol synthesize cell surface receptors (LDL receptor) that recognize apoprotein B specifically. Within 10 min of binding, the LDL particle is internalized and delivered to the lysosomes, where the cholesterol is released from the cholesterol esters. LDL receptors are localized in clusters over small indentations or pits with a bristle-like appearance, termed **coated pits**. The coated pits invaginate and pinch off from the plasma membrane to form **coated vesicles** (Fig. 4.29). This constitutive membrane invagination results in the internalization of receptors in coated pits whether or not they are occupied by ligand. Coated vesicles are quickly uncoated and the uncoated vesicles then fuse with larger smooth vesicles called **endosomes**. The pH of the endosome is maintained between approximately 5.5 and 6.0 by an **ATP-dependent proton pump**. At this pH the LDL receptor has a low affinity for the LDL particle and the two dissociate. The endosome is also known as the **C**ompartment for the **U**ncoupling of **R**eceptor and **L**igand (**CURL**). The transmembranous receptors are sequestered to a domain within the endosome membrane that buds off as a vesicle and recycles the LDL receptor to the plasma membrane. Recycled receptors are inserted randomly in the plasma membrane but are quickly sequestered again into coated pits. The contents of the endosome are passed on to lysosomes such that the cholesterol esters can be hydrolysed and released into the cell. Whether this involves fusion of endosomes and lysosomes or the passage of transport vesicles between compartments remains to be resolved. Thus, the LDLs and their receptors are sorted from each other in the endosome.

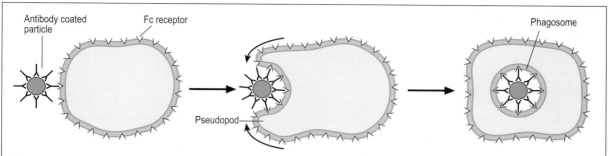

Fig. 4.27 Phagocytosis of antibody-coated particles by macrophages and neutrophils. Sequential binding of receptors guides surrounding pseudopods.

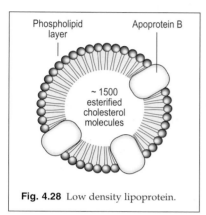

Fig. 4.28 Low density lipoprotein.

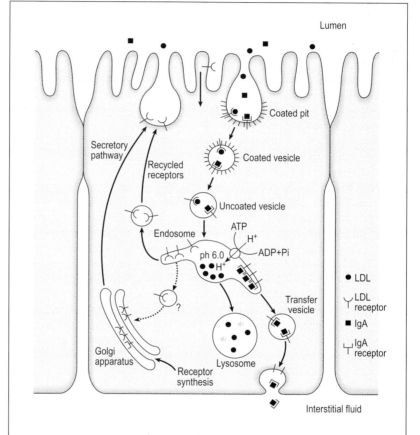

Fig. 4.29 Receptor-mediated endocytosis. Compartments are drawn as distinct vesicular structures. Whether this is the case or whether these structures form parts of an interconnecting tubular system is still debated. There is some evidence for exchange of components between the endocytic and secretory pathways.

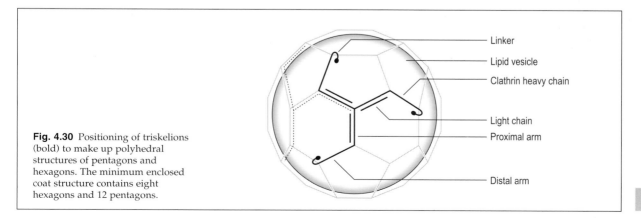

Fig. 4.30 Positioning of triskelions (bold) to make up polyhedral structures of pentagons and hexagons. The minimum enclosed coat structure contains eight hexagons and 12 pentagons.

4

Coat structure

The association of the coat proteins is energy-independent and, therefore, coated-pit formation is spontaneous. The minimum structure that can be formed is a three-legged structure called the **triskelion**, containing **clathrin** and two **light chains** in the ratio 3 : 2 : 1 (Fig. 4.30). It is proposed that the triskelions associate to form a basket-like structure consisting of hexagons and pentagons (Fig. 4.30). Because assembly is spontaneous, uncoating must be driven. This is carried out by an ATP-dependent uncoating protein which binds and stabilizes the freed coat proteins. The clathrin coat is attached to the plasma membrane by several integral membrane adapter proteins. These proteins form associations with both the clathrin and the receptors, locating the receptors over the coated pit.

Four modes of receptor-mediated endocytosis

Receptors for different ligands enter the cell via the same coated pits and the pathway from coated pits to the endosome is common for all proteins that undergo endocytosis. In addition to **mode 1**, exemplified by LDL/LDL receptor uptake, different modes of this process can be defined on the basis of the destination of internalized receptor and ligand (Table 4.2). Receptors targeted to different cellular destinations, by short amino acid motifs, are sorted within the CURL to discrete regions of membrane, which bud-off into transport vesicles.

Mode 2: uptake of ferric (Fe^{3+}) ions by **transferrin**. Two ferric ions (Fe^{3+}) bind to apotransferrin, forming transferrin in the circulation. Transferrin (but not apotransferrin, which only has a low affinity for the receptor) binds to the transferrin receptor and is internalized as above. On reaching the acidic endosome, the Fe^{3+} is released from the transferrin but at this pH the apotransferrin has an increased affinity for the receptor and remains associated. The complex is sorted in the CURL for recycling back to the plasma membrane, where, at pH 7.4, the apotransferrin dissociates from the transferrin receptor again.

Mode 3: uptake of occupied **insulin receptors**. Most receptors involved in receptor-mediated endocytosis are located over the coated pits, but some, such as the insulin receptor, only congregate over the coated pits when insulin is bound. Insulin binding probably induces a conformational change in the insulin receptor that allows it to be recognized by the coated pit. In the endosome, insulin remains bound to the receptor and the complex is targeted to the lysosomes for degradation via **multivesicular bodies**. These structures accumulate small membrane vesicles derived from the perimeter membrane, thereby completely internalizing the receptor. This mechanism allows for the reduction in the number of insulin receptors on the membrane surface (down-regulation) which **desensitizes** the cell to a continued presence of high circulating insulin concentrations.

Mode 4: transcytosis. Some ligands that remain bound to their receptors may be transported across the cell, e.g. maternal immunoglobulins to the fetus via the placenta, transfer of immunoglobulin A (IgA) from the circulation to bile in the liver. During transport of IgA the receptor is cleaved, resulting in the release of immunoglobulin with a bound 'secretory component' derived from the receptor.

Mode	Fate of receptor	Fate of ligand	Examples	Function
1	Recycled	Degraded	LDL	Metabolite uptake
2	Recycled	Recycled	Transferrin	Metabolite uptake
3	Degraded	Degraded	Insulin, Epidermal growth factor,	Receptor down-regulation
			Immune complexes	Removal from circulation of foreign antigen
4	Transported	Transported	Maternal IgG Secretory IgA	Transfer of large molecules across the cell.

Table 4.2 Destinations of receptors and ligands taken up by receptor-mediated endocytosis

Mutations affecting the LDL receptor in hypercholesterolaemia

Naturally occurring mutations of the LDL receptor have been identified in some patients with **hypercholesterolaemia**. Three mutations, when found in a homozygous individual, lead to three phenotypes:

1. *Non-functional receptor*. The LDL receptor is unable to bind LDL. However, the receptors cluster over normal coated pits and are internalized.
2. *Functional receptor binding only 10% of normal LDL*. Normal internalization occurs but the efficiency of LDL uptake is reduced by the reduced affinity of binding to the receptor.
3. *Receptor binding normal*. No internalization of bound LDL occurs because of a deletion in the C-terminal of the receptor that makes the interaction with the coated pits. In these patients, LDL receptors are found distributed over the whole cell surface rather than clustered over coated pits.

Treatment of hypercholesterolaemia

Hypercholesterolaemia is a risk factor for cardiovascular complications due to deposition of cholesterol on the vasculature. Lowering of cholesterol levels may be achieved by modification of lipoprotein metabolism, by altered diet, the use of bile acid sequestrant resins (to increase excretion), statins (hydroxymethylglutaryl coenzyme A reductase inhibitors to inhibit cholesterol synthesis) or fibrates (activators of lipoprotein lipase that reduce triglyceride levels and also increase LDL uptake by LDL receptors).

Viruses and toxins

Membrane-enveloped viruses and some toxins exploit endocytic pathways to enter cells after binding to receptors in the plasma membrane. Once in the endosome, where the acid pH is favourable, the viral membrane is able to fuse with the endosomal membrane, thereby releasing the viral RNA into the cell where it can be translated and replicated to form new viral particles.

Further reading

Decamilli P, Emr S D, McPherson P S, Novick P 1996 Phosphoinositides as regulators in membrane traffic. Science 271: 1533–1539

Houslay M D, Stanley K K 1984 Dynamics of biological membranes: influence on synthesis, structure and function. John Wiley and Sons, Chichester

Jay D G 1996 Role of band-3 in homeostasis and cell-shape. Cell 86: 853–854

Rothman J E, Wieland F T 1996 Protein sorting by transport vesicles. Science 272: 227–234

Schekman R, Orci I 1996 Coat proteins and vesicle budding. Science 271: 1526–1533

Revision questions

1. Outline the common features of biological membranes. What are the functions of the plasma membrane of cells?

2. What is the function of cholesterol in the plasma membrane?

3. What modes of mobility are permitted for membrane lipids and proteins? How may the mobility of membrane proteins be restricted in cells?

4. What is the difference between passive and active transport across membranes?

5. What is the difference between primary and secondary active transport?

6. In what ways can membrane transport contribute (a) to the regulation of cell volume and (b) the regulation of intracellular pH?

7. In receptor-mediated endocytosis how are (a) the invagination of the plasma membrane, (b) the uncoating of coated vesicles and (c) the uncoupling of receptor and ligand achieved? In what ways do cells make use of receptor-mediated endocytosis? How may viruses take advantages of this process?

Answers to revision questions

1. Biological membranes are composed of a dynamic phospholipid bilayer, studded with various integral membrane proteins and associated with various peripheral membrane proteins. The plasma membrane isolates cellular contents from their environment, controls the movement of substances and thereby permits control of the intracellular environment. It mediates direct communication between cells and within cells in response to extracellular signals.

2. The function of cholesterol in the plasma membrane is to stabilize the membrane bilayer.

3. Membrane lipids and proteins may undergo vibrational, rotational and lateral movements within the membrane bilayer. Phospholipids may also undergo flip-flop. The mobility of membrane proteins may be restricted by attachment to cytoskeletal elements within the cell or to extracellular molecules, either in the extracellular matrix or on adjacent cells.

4. Passive transport occurs when transport down an electrochemical gradient is thermodynamically favourable. Active transport requires the input of energy from a thermodynamically favourable reaction to move the transported species against an unfavourable electrochemical gradient.

5. Primary active transport is coupled directly to ATP hydrolysis to provide the energy to drive transport. Secondary active transport is coupled to the concentration gradient of another ionic or molecular species to provide the energy for transport.

6. (a) Using the electrochemical Na^+ gradient generated by the Na^+–K^+ ATPase, cells may respond to cell swelling by extruding K^+ and Cl^- via channels, co-transporters or coupled to the uptake of HCO_3^- to reduce cytoplasmic osmotic strength (see Fig. 4.25). In response to shrinking, cells respond to increase cytoplasmic ionic strength by increasing Na^+, Cl^- and sometimes K^+ concentration via Na^+–K^+–$2Cl^-$ co-transport, Na^+–Cl^- co-transport and Na^+–H^+ and anion exchange (see Fig. 4.25). (b) Using the electrochemical Na^+ gradient, cells may drive proton extrusion via Na^+–H^+ exchange and in some cells Na^+–Cl^-–HCO_3^-–H^+ co-transport. Cells may also use Na^+–HCO_3^- co-transport to take up HCO_3^- to reduce cell acidity. Most cells possess an anion exchanger to permit the movement of HCO_3^- buffer.

7. (a) Invagination of the membrane occurs by the spontaneous formation of basket-like clathrin coat structures on the cytoplasmic surface of the plasma membrane. (b) Uncoating of coated vesicles is mediated by an uncoating protein, which uses ATP hydrolysis to provide the energy to overcome the unfavourable thermodynamics of the process. (c) Uncoupling of receptors and ligands occurs in endosomes (CURL) when binding affinity is reduced as a result of the acidity in this compartment. Cells use receptor-mediated endocytosis for the specific uptake of metabolites and proteins, cell desensitization and the transport of macromolecules across the cell. Some membrane-bound viruses can take advantage of the process, following receptor binding and internalization, because of membrane fusion that occurs at the pH of the endosome, which releases the viral genome into the cytoplasm for replication.

Organelles: compartmentalization of cellular functions and protein targeting

Organelles with double membranes

Nucleus

Under the microscope the most prominent organelle in all eukaryotic cells (with the exception of erythrocytes) is the nucleus (Fig. 5.1). The nucleus compartmentalizes reactions involving the synthesis of DNA, RNA and ribonuclear protein complexes. This separates nuclear mRNA transcription from cytoplasmic translation into protein, which, in turn, permits post-transcriptional processing of mRNA and an additional level of complexity in the organization and expression of the genetic code.

In non-dividing cells (interphase) each nucleus contains two complete copies of the genomic DNA, which is packaged into **chromosomes**. The chromosomal complement or **karyotype** of normal human males and females is 22 homologous pairs of chromosomes plus the Y and X sex chromosomes, respectively. A sub-organelle of the nucleus that is seen by microscopy is the **nucleolus**, in which new ribosomes are assembled. Nucleoli are **nucleoprotein** complexes of protein, RNA and regions of several chromosomes encoding ribosomal components called collectively the **nucleolar organizer**. The nuclear contents in the **nucleoplasm** are surrounded by a double layer of membrane, which makes up the **nuclear envelope**. The outer membrane is contiguous with the rough endoplasmic reticulum (ER) and may bear ribosomes involved in the synthesis of nuclear components. Some of these nascent proteins are translocated into the space between the inner and outer nuclear membrane, termed the **periplasmic** or **perinuclear space**, which forms a continuum of the ER lumen. The structure of the nucleus is determined by the **nuclear lamina**, a dense network of rod-like **lamin neurofilaments** that forms associations between DNA molecules and the inner membrane.

Chromatin

In non-dividing cells the single molecule of double-stranded DNA that comprises each chromosome is packaged into a dense and highly organized supercoiled structure of DNA, protein and some RNA called **chromatin** (Fig. 5.2). In non-dividing cells in interphase, the highly condensed form, termed **heterochromatin**, is localized around the periphery of the nucleus and nucleolus in association with the nuclear lamina. For gene transcription and replication the heterochromatin structure must be unravelled. In interphase approximately 10% of the chromatin is in the unwound form (**euchromatin**) where active RNA transcription is taking place.

Nuclear pores

Communication between the nucleoplasm and cytoplasm is mediated exclusively by selective **nuclear pore** structures which punctuate the nuclear envelope (Fig. 5.3). These nuclear pores allow the uninhibited two-way passage of small molecules and proteins up to a molecular weight of ~60 kDa (~9 nm diameter). However, nuclear proteins much larger than this cut-off size can pass through the nuclear pores following synthesis in the cytoplasm, as can preformed ribosomal complexes and mRNA passing into the cytoplasm. The selective transport of large molecules is receptor-mediated, requiring recognition of nuclear targeting signal motifs by the nuclear pore complex. Several short primary sequences that target proteins to the nucleus have been identified but no common structural similarity exists between them, suggesting that a family of receptor proteins for different signals must be involved. The selective transport process is also energy-dependent. In the absence of ATP, import of nuclear proteins is inhibited even though the proteins cluster over the nuclear pore complexes.

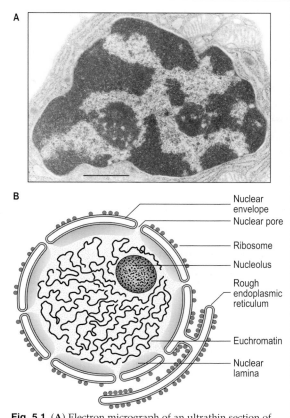

Fig. 5.1 (**A**) Electron micrograph of an ultrathin section of a nucleus. Bar = 1 micron. (**B**) Schematic diagram of a typical cell nucleus in interphase. (EM courtesy of Mrs Evaline Roberts and Dr Arthur J. Rowe)

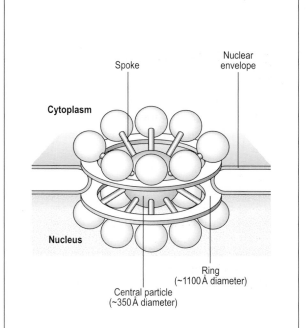

Fig. 5.3 Model of the structure of a nuclear pore. The pore structure (100 nm diameter) is made up of an octamer of protein subunits which line a pore of ~10 nm. In some preparations, the pore is plugged by a central granule protein. The components that form the pore structures and the mechanism of transport, particularly of ribosomal complexes that are larger than the apparent pore diameter, remain to be elucidated.

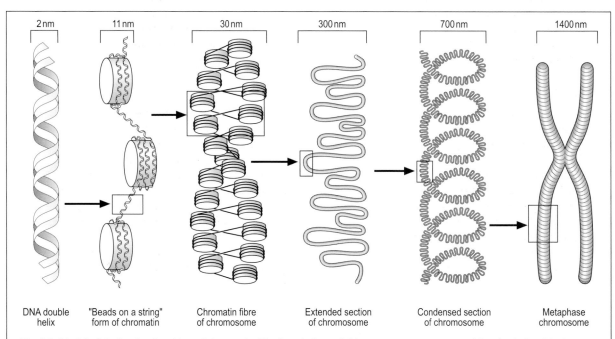

Fig. 5.2 Model of the levels of packing of chromatin. The foundations of this structure are octamers of four basic (positively charged), highly conserved proteins called **histones** (two copies each of H2a, H2b, H3 and H4). Lengths (~145 base pairs) of the double stranded DNA molecule are wound twice around each histone octamer to form a **nucleosome**. The highly positive core stabilizes the negatively charged DNA molecule. Successive nucleosomes are separated by short lengths (40–100 base pairs) of internucleosomal DNA. This condensation forms the first level of chromatin structure, the **10 nm fibre**. The next level of structure, the **30 nm fibre**, is stabilized by a fifth histone, H1, which binds to the nucleosome and, by cooperative H1–H1 interactions, draws adjacent nucleosomes together. Loops in this structure form a higher order **300 nm fibre** which can coil further into **700 nm fibres**.

Mitochondria

The primary function of mitochondria (Fig. 5.4) is to provide the machinery for oxidative phosphorylation to allow the efficient release of energy from catabolism of fuel molecules and the concomitant production of ATP (Fig. 5.5). Enzymes of the major metabolic pathways are located in the matrix while the components of the electron transport chain and oxidative phosphorylation are all located on the cristae formed from the inner mitochondrial membrane. The inner membrane is essentially impermeable to protons. The outer mitochondrial membrane is punctuated with transmembranous **porin** pores, which allows the passage of proteins up to ~ 10 kDa. Thus, for small molecules and protons the intermembrane space is essentially continuous with the cytoplasm.

The mitochondrial genome

As organelles, mitochondria are exceptional in that they possess several copies of a small circular DNA genome of their own and produce some of their own polypeptides. Small differences in the genetic code employed are found in the mitochondrial genome (mitochondrial/universal codes: AGA, Stop/Arg; AGG, Stop/Arg; AUA, Met/Ile; UGA, Trp/Stop). The genome encodes just two mitochondrial ribosomal RNAs, 22 transfer RNAs and 13 subunit components of the electron transport/oxidative phosphorylation complexes, so most of the mitochondrial proteins are encoded by the nuclear genome and must be targeted to the mitochondrion.

Diseases mediated by mitochondrial genes

Mutations in the mitochondrial genome can lead to weakness in skeletal (myopathy) and cardiac (cardiomyopathy) muscle, as well as systemic problems associated with nervous system disorders such as ataxia (staggering gait), myoclonus (uncontrolled jerking movement), epilepsy and dementia. In many cases there is little relationship between the mutation and specific clinical features, although there are some exceptions (Table 5.1). Severity of a mitochondrial gene-mediated disease may be reduced by the presence of non-defective mitochondria, so-called **heteroplasmy**.

Mitochondira grow and divide during the non-dividing phase of the cell cycle (interphase) and are shared between daughter cells on cell division. Because most mitochondrial proteins are encoded in the nucleus, most mitochondrial diseases are inherited in a Mendelian fashion. However, because sperm only contribute nuclear material to the ovum at fertilization, mutations in mitochondrially encoded proteins have a maternal pattern of inheritance.

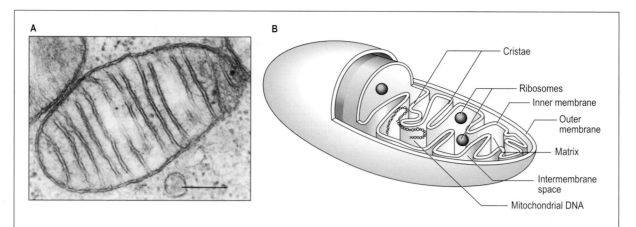

Fig. 5.4 (**A**) Electron micrograph of an ultrathin section of mitochondrion. Bar = 200 nm. (**B**) Schematic diagram of a mitochondrion sectioned to show its contents. (EM courtesy of Mrs Evaline Roberts and Dr Arthur J. Rowe)

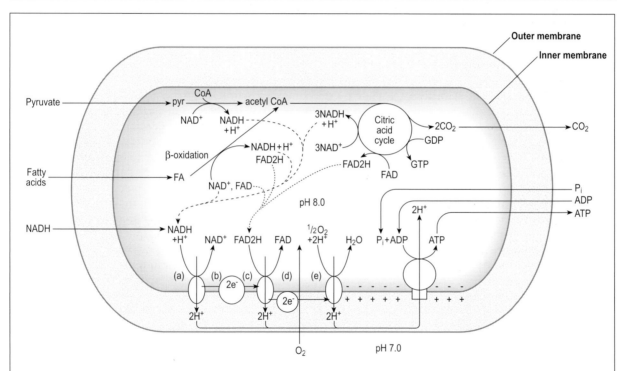

Fig. 5.5 The major metabolic functions of mitochondria. Mitochondria contain the enzymes of the citric acid cycle and fatty acid β-oxidation pathways both of which efficiently pass the reducing potential from substrates to the electron and hydrogen carriers, NADH and FAD2H. Reoxidation of these carriers by molecular oxygen, catalysed in a stepwise fashion by the electron transport chain, converts the chemical reducing potential into an electrochemical potential (~ −160 mV) across the mitochondrial inner membrane by extruding a proton (H^+) from the mitochondrion each time an electron carrier protein changes conformation as it passes on the electron down the chain. Protons in the cytoplasm experience an electrochemical driving force favouring re-entry into the mitochondrion composed of (1) the electrical potential and (2) the chemical gradient that results from the alkalization of the mitochondrial matrix to ~pH 8.0 (relative to the cytosolic pH of ~7.0), which occurs as the protons are extruded from the organelle. Dissipation of the electrochemical gradient by re-entry of protons through the ATP synthetase provides the energy for the synthesis of ATP from ADP and P_i. a, NADH dehydrogenase; b, ubiquinone, c, b1-c complex; d, cytochrome c; e, cytochrome oxidase.

Gene affected	Disease
ATPase 6	Neurogenic disorders, weakness, retinitis pigmentosa, Leigh's disease
Cytochrome c oxidase	Floppy baby syndrome, respiratory distress treated with high oxygen
ND1 or ND6	Leber's hereditary optic neuropathy (LHON), sudden irreversible blindness, prevalent in young males
tRNA *leu*	Myoclonus, encephalopathy with stroke-like episodes (MELAS)
tRNA *lys*	Myoclonus, epilepsy with ragged fibres (MERRP)
	Uncontrolled and irregular eye movements

Table 5.1 Mitochondrial protein mutations leading to specific genetic defects

Organelles with single membranes

Endoplasmic reticulum

Functions of the endoplasmic reticulum

The ER is composed of a network of flattened sacs and tubules of membrane, termed **cisternae**, all of which interconnect to form a common lumen. In muscle tissue the ER is termed the **sarcoplasmic reticulum (SR)**. This membrane structure may represent up to half of the total cell membrane in an actively secreting cell. It forms a continuation of the nuclear envelope such that the ER lumen is continuous with the periplasmic space of the nuclear envelope and is often arranged in concentric flattened layers around the nucleus. The association of **ribosomes** with the ER allows a region of **rough ER** to be distinguished from areas of **smooth ER** devoid of ribosomal contacts. Ribosomes associated with rough ER are actively involved in the synthesis of secretory, lysosomal and membrane proteins.

Other functions of the ER include the synthesis of membrane lipids, phospholipids (Fig. 5.6), steroids and triglycerides and functions involving electron transport activities such as the introduction of double bonds into fatty acids by the cytochrome b_5 electron transport chain and detoxification of cellular toxins and drugs by the cytochrome P_{450} electron transfer system. The ER is also important for the maintenance of low $[Ca^{2+}]_i$ (see Fig. 7.7) and is an important source of Ca^{2+} that can be mobilized for intracellular signalling (see Figs 7.8 and 7.9).

Secretory and membrane protein biosynthesis

Like cytosolic proteins, membrane proteins and those to be secreted or targeted to lysosomes are synthesized against the mRNA template by ribosomes. However, before synthesis progresses very far the translation of these proteins is halted until the ribosome has been transferred to the rough ER (Fig. 5.7). A characteristic hydrophobic amino acid sequence of 18–30 amino acids flanked by basic residues at the N-terminus of the nascent polypeptide, termed the **signal** or **leader** sequence, is recognized by a large protein/RNA complex called the **signal recognition particle (SRP)**. Binding of the SRP to the growing polypeptide chain and the ribosome locks the ribosome complex and prevents further protein synthesis while the ribosome is in the cytoplasm.

On the ER the SRP is recognized by an **SRP receptor** or **docking protein**. In making the interaction with the docking protein, the SRP is released from the signal sequence of the nascent polypeptide removing the inhibitory constraint on further translation. The signal sequence then interacts with a **signal sequence receptor (SSR)** in the ER membrane, which directs further synthesis through the ER membrane. The ribosome becomes anchored by **ribophorin** proteins. The ribophorins, possibly together with the SSR, are thought to form the pore through which the growing polypeptide chain is extruded. In the case of a secreted or lysosomal protein, synthesis is completed and the nascent protein is translocated into the lumen of the ER. For membrane proteins the passage of the protein through the membrane must be arrested. The **stop-transfer signal** for this is a highly hydrophobic primary sequence in the growing polypeptide of between 18 and 22 amino acids long followed directly by charged amino acids which, in α-helical form, is long enough to span the hydrophobic core of the bilayer. This sequence forms the transmembranous region of the protein. The ribosome then presumably detaches from the ER and protein biosynthesis continues in the cytoplasm. The result is a transmembrane protein with its N-terminal directed into the lumen and its C-terminal to the cytoplasm. For both secretory proteins and membrane incorporated proteins the signal sequence is cleaved from the new protein by **signal peptidases** even before protein synthesis is completed.

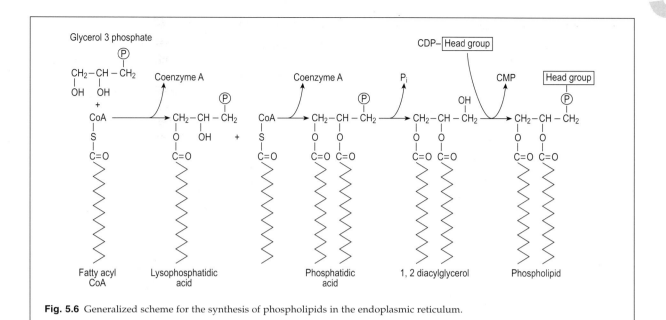

Fig. 5.6 Generalized scheme for the synthesis of phospholipids in the endoplasmic reticulum.

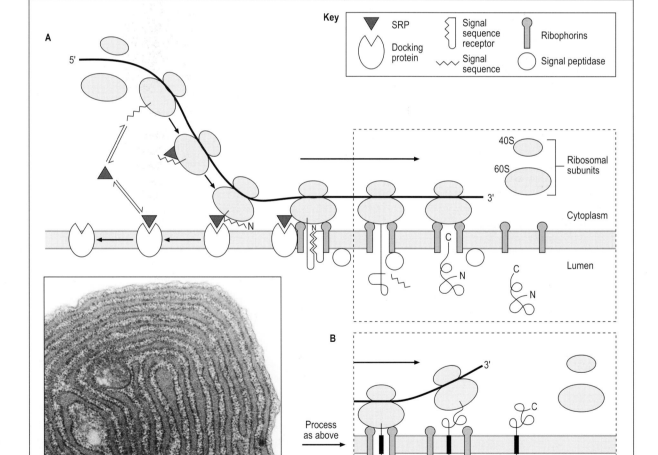

Fig. 5.7 (**A**) Secretory and (**B**) membrane protein biosynthesis on rough endoplasmic reticulum. *Inset*: electron micrograph of an ultrathin section of rough endoplasmic reticulum. Bar = 1 micron. (EM courtesy of Mrs Evaline Roberts and Dr Arthur J. Rowe)

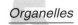

Membrane insertion of proteins with multiple membrane-spanning domains

Where a protein has multiple transmembrane domains it is likely that the folding of the nascent protein against the constraint of the first transmembrane segment is the driving force for the insertion of the other domains (Fig. 5.8A). This is unlikely to be a simple process and the mechanisms underlying the insertion of multiple transmembrane domain proteins remain to be determined. It is possible that a series of start- and stop-tranfer sequences within the primary structure control membrane insertion. The association of lumenal binding proteins (e.g. BiP) related to the family of heat-shock proteins (hsp) also assists in stabilizing the partially folded growing polypeptide.

Strategies for alternative membrane topology

Where a mature membrane protein presents its N-terminal on the cytoplasmic side of the membrane it is thought that the signal sequence may be contained within the primary structure of the growing polypeptide rather than at the N-terminal and that it may correspond to the first transmembrane domain (Fig. 5.8B). In this case the emerging loop of C-terminal sequence in the ER lumen must be resistant to signal peptidase cleavage. Multispanning topologies can follow as before. Whatever the final topology of a mature membrane protein, it is protein synthesis that directs their asymmetrical orientation (Figs 5.7 and 5.8).

Insertion of membrane proteins synthesized in the cytoplasm

It is noteworthy that a few proteins synthesized totally in the cytoplasm, including all mitochondrial proteins, can be inserted post-translationally into membranes by an ATP-driven process (Fig. 5.8C). Insertion of folded proteins is thermodynamically most unfavourable and, hence, this process most likely requires that proteins for post-translational insertion be unfolded. Stabilizing proteins related to the **hsp 70 heat shock protein** family (**chaperonins**) and tunnel-forming proteins in the membrane are likely to be involved but these remain to be identified. Alternatively, some proteins become membrane anchored via a post-translational covalent addition of a hydrocarbon chain (palmityolation, mystriolation), which binds the protein to a single leaflet of the membrane bilayer (Fig. 5.8D).

Protein incorporation into mitochondria

The mitochondrial protein signal sequence is located generally in the N-terminal 20–80 residues, which coil to form an amphipathic α-helix with non-polar residues on one face and positively charged residues on the other. Unlike the ER, where transmembrane movement of the protein occurs co-translationally, uptake of protein into the mitochondrion occurs post-translationally. Therefore, on binding of the signal sequence to a receptor protein in the outer membrane, the protein must be unfolded to allow the vectorial movement of protein across the membrane.

The details of mitochondrial protein uptake remain to be elucidated but protein translocation is known to be ATP-dependent and involves a member of the hsp 70 heat shock family of proteins to stabilize the unfolded proteins as they are translocated. Models for the targeting of proteins within the mitochondrion depend on the positioning of start-transfer and stop-transfer signals in the primary structure of the protein (Fig. 5.9). Transfer of mitochondrial proteins occurs at specific adhesion sites between the inner and outer membrane such that insertion of the signal sequence initiates vectorial transfer. Once in the mitochondrial matrix the signal sequence is removed by a signal peptidase and the transported protein folds into its mature structure. The transfer of outer membrane proteins is arrested by stop-transfer sequences within the primary sequence. Proteins that are located in the inner mitochondrial membrane or the intermembrane space are thought to be targeted back to the inner membrane by a start-transfer sequence that is revealed on cleavage of the signal sequence from the translocated protein. The mechanism is analogous to that in the ER such that the start-transfer signal of intermembrane proteins binds to a receptor followed by the complete passage of the protein through the membrane. Cleavage of the start-transfer signal by a specific protease releases the protein into the intermembranous space. Insertion of inner membrane proteins probably occurs by the same process except that translocation is arrested by stop-transfer sequences. As in the ER, multiple transmembrane spanning proteins are probably located by a series of start- and stop-transfer sequences.

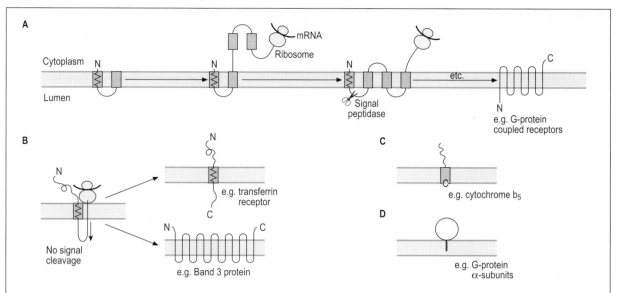

Fig. 5.8 Models of the strategies for the production of membrane proteins with alternative topography. Cleavage of the signal sequence by signal peptidase results in proteins with a lumenally directed N-terminus (**A**). Where no signal cleavage occurs, the N-terminal is directed towards the cytoplasm (**B**). Some proteins may also be inserted into the membrane post-translationally either via a hydrophobic sequence within the protein (**C**) or following the post-translational covalent addition of a hydrocarbon moiety (**D**). c, cytoplasm; l, lumen of the endoplasmic reticulum.

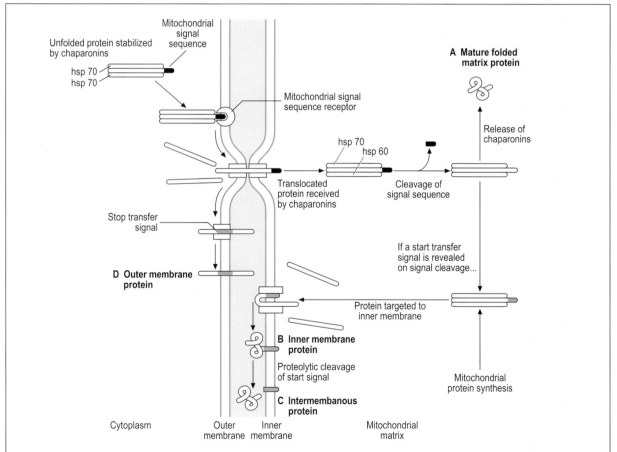

Fig. 5.9 Models for the targeting and incorporation of mitochondrial proteins synthesized in the cytoplasm. N-terminal mitochondrial targeting sequences direct proteins to the mitochondrial protein import mechanism. Translocated matrix proteins are probably stabilized by mitochondrial chaperonins before folding into the mature structure (**A**). If a start transfer signal is revealed on cleavage of the mitochondrial signal sequence, an internalized protein is redirected to the inner membrane where it incorporates (**B**). Cleavage of intermembranously oriented polypeptide by matrix proteases releases intermembranous proteins (**C**). Outer membrane protein may be located by stop-transfer signals which prevent full translocation of a mitochondrially-targeted protein (**D**).

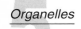

Post-translational modification of secretory and membrane proteins

In addition to signal peptide cleavage, post-translational modifications to secretory and membrane proteins such as disulphide bond formation (Fig. 5.10), glycosylation (Fig. 5.11) and proteolytic modification (see Fig. 5.13) are commenced as soon as the amino acid to bear the modification appears in the lumen of the ER. The nascent chain is further processed as it passes from the ER and through the cis- to trans-Golgi. The new protein continues along the **secretory pathway** until the secretory vesicle fuses with the plasma membrane. At this point, secreted proteins are released from the cell and membrane proteins are delivered such that the regions of the protein that were located in the cytoplasm during synthesis remain with this orientation.

The Golgi apparatus

The cis-, medial- and trans-Golgi are functionally distinct regions of the Golgi apparatus and are distinguished by the specific localization of different enzymes within them. Sequential passage of newly synthesized polypeptide chains from cis- to trans-Golgi regions provides a mechanism for an ordered series of post-translational modifications.

Protein glycosylation

Unlike proteins translated in the cytoplasm, most proteins synthesized on the ER become post-translationally modified on their lumenal aspect by the addition of complex carbohydrate chains. This glycosylation can be N-linked to the amino side-chain group on asparagine residues (Fig. 5.11) or O-linked to the hydroxyl group of serine, threonine and, in collagen, hydroxylysine. The nature of the final oligosaccharide modification is governed by the conformation of the protein, the information for which is contained within the primary sequence. All glycoprotein modifications are directed to the extracytoplasmic face of cellular membranes.

N-linked glycosylation occurs specifically on asparagine residues in the sequence Asn-X-Ser or Asn-X-Thr, where X is any amino acid except proline. N-linked glycosylation is initiated in the lumen of the ER by the transfer by an oligosaccharide-protein transferase of a presynthesized oligomer of 14 sugar units from a carrier lipid called dolichol phosphate. Glucose residues are then removed to reveal a high mannose core, which is then further modified as the protein passes through the ER and Golgi apparatus (summarized in Fig. 5.11).

O-linked glycosylation is initiated through the direct action of glycosyl transferases on the protein and complex oligosaccharide chains are then built up.

Function of protein glycosylation

Glycosylation is important for the native structure and function of some proteins, protects others from premature degradation, and in others appears to have no beneficial effect. In some proteins the nature of the carbohydrate modification influences the targeting of proteins to their cellular location.

Non-specific protein glycosylation in diabetes mellitus

An exception to the absence of glycosylation of cytoplasmic proteins is the non-specific glycosylation of these proteins that occurs spontaneously in hyperglycaemia. Such non-specific glycosylation can be detrimental to protein function and in diabetes mellitus underlies many of the secondary microvascular complications in this disease. Clinical measurement of the level of glycosylated haemoglobin (HbA$_{1c}$) is used as a measure of overall glycaemic control.

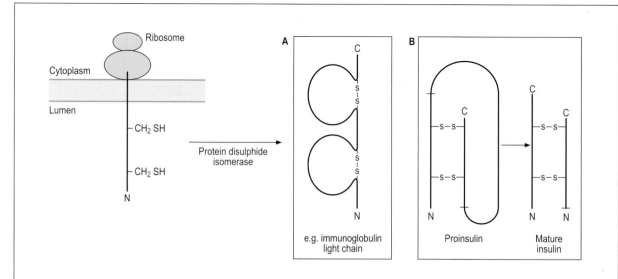

Fig. 5.10 Protein disulphide isomerase (PDI) catalyses the introduction of 'correct' disulphide bonds into new proteins either (**A**) during synthesis or (**B**) as a post-translational modification. This can result in the disulphide linkage of sequential cysteine residues in the primary sequence (**A**) but is not the case for all proteins (**B**). PDI is not required absolutely for disulphide bond formation in the oxidizing environment of the ER lumen but this enzyme probably constrains stable protein conformations in nascent proteins to ensure the formation of 'correct' disulphide bridges. c, cytoplasm; l, lumen.

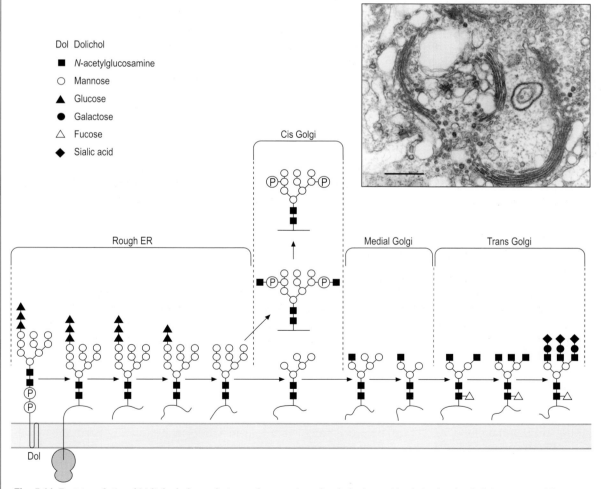

Fig. 5.11 Post-translational N-linked glycosylation and processing of carbohydrate side chains by the Golgi apparatus. New sugar residues are added in the Golgi apparatus by glycosyl transferases from uridine diphosphate (UDP)-activated sugars. *Inset*: electron micrograph of Golgi apparatus. Bar = 1 micron. (EM courtesy of Mrs Evaline Roberts and Dr Arthur J. Rowe)

Lysosomal targeting via mannose 6-phosphate residues

Rather than receive a complex oligosaccharide modification, the high mannose cores of oligosaccharide chains on enzymes targeted to a lysosomal localization are phosphorylated in the cis-Golgi to mannose 6-phosphate. Phosphorylated mannose serves as the signal for lysosomal targeting by binding to a mannose 6-phosphate receptor (at neutral pH) in the trans-Golgi, which directs the proteins to acidic sorting vesicles (Fig. 5.12). These vesicles may be synonymous with CURL (see Chapter 4) and the acidic pH may release the enzymes into the lumen, allowing the receptor to recycle to the Golgi apparatus and vesicles containing the lysosomal enzymes to be directed to their lysosomal destination. The action of phosphatases may also prevent rebinding of the enzymes with their receptors in this compartment.

Lysosomal storage diseases

Mutations in lysosomal enzymes that result in loss of function or abnormal targeting to the lysosome give rise to a large number of lysosomal storage diseases with overlapping phenotypes. The inability to digest various substrates causes lysosomes to swell, leading to a wide range of dysfunction in different tissues. For example:

- A mutation in β-N-acetylhexosaminidase in **Tay-Sachs' disease** results in accumulation of ganglioside G_{M2} in children leading to dementia and blindness.
- Defective β-glucuronidase in **Sly syndrome** results in abnormal lysosomes in many tissues due to the inability to breakdown proteoglycan.
- **Inclusion cell (I-cell) disease** occurs because of inappropriate sorting of lysosomal enzymes for export, due to the absence of mannose 6-phosphate residues in carbohydrate side chains which target lysosomal enzymes. Large undigested inclusion bodies form in the lysosomes of these patients who develop severe skeletal deformities and psychomotor deficiencies. Treatment of fibroblasts from I-cell disease patients with lysosomal proteins bearing mannose 6-phosphate restores a normal appearance to the cells (Fig. 5.12). Such treatments could provide a potential mechanism for the treatment of other lysosomal storage diseases where individual proteins are defective such as **Hurler's syndrome** (α-iduronidase) and Tay-Sachs' disease.

Post-translational proteolysis

Many polypeptides are produced as larger proproteins from which the active polypeptide is cleaved by proteolysis. Often this proteolysis occurs on the C-terminal side of a pair of basic residues, after which the two basic residues are themselves removed. Proteolysis to release the active species often occurs late in the maturation of the protein to avoid unwanted intracellular effects. For example, lysosomal hydrolase enzymes are made as inactive proenzymes and are only activated in the lysosomal compartment by proteases that are active in an acidic environment, thus protecting the contents of the ER and Golgi apparatus. Similarly, insulin is only processed from the proinsulin precursor in the secretory vesicle (Fig. 5.10B). This prevents inappropriate activation of insulin receptors that may be present in the ER compartment. The acid pH in the secretory vesicle restricts any binding of insulin to receptors that may be present in the secretory granule. Post-translational proteolysis also provides a mechanism for the release of multiple copies of a hormone from a single prohormone molecule, e.g. five copies of the pituitary hormone methionine-enkephalin (Tyr-Gly-Gly-Phe-Met) and one copy of leucine-enkephalin (Tyr-Gly-Gly-Phe-Leu) are released from a single prohormone molecule. Alternatively, multiple active hormone species may be produced from a single prohormone species, e.g. cleavage of pro-opiomelanocorticotrophin (POMC) in the anterior and intermediate lobes of the pituitary results in the production of adrenocorticotrophic hormone (ACTH), β-lipotrophin (β-LPH), γ-lipotrophin (γ-LPH), β-endorphin and other hormones (Fig. 5.13). In the intermediate lobe, ACTH can be processed further to α-melanocyte-stimulating hormone (α-MSH) and corticotrophin-like intermediate lobe peptide (CLIP). In this case, post-translational proteolysis allows for the concerted release of hormone molecules with different tissue targets and, indeed, for different mixtures of hormones depending on the tissue of origin.

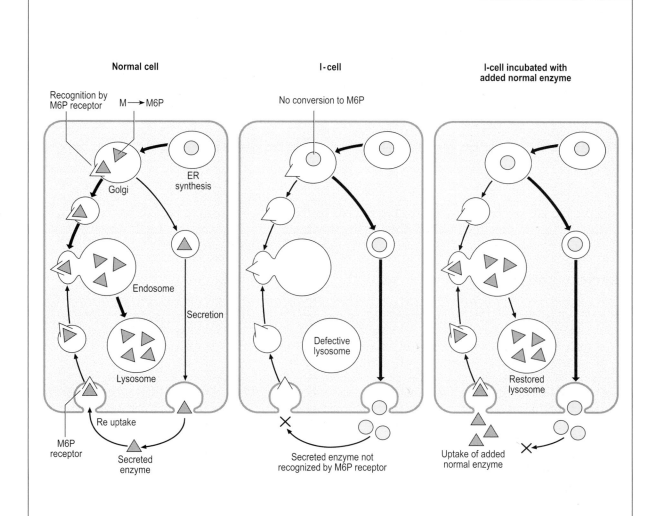

Fig. 5.12 Targeting of lysosomal enzymes in normal cells and I-cell disease. Circles represent mannose and triangles represent mannose-6-phosphate in core oligosaccharide. Bold arrows show the route taken by newly synthesized lysosomal enzymes. UDP-N-acetylglucosamine phosphotransferase shows specificity for a recognition site on lysosomal enzyme precursors. This ensures that other glycosylated proteins are not misdirected to lysosomes. Note: this enzyme uses an 'activated' nucleotide sugar.

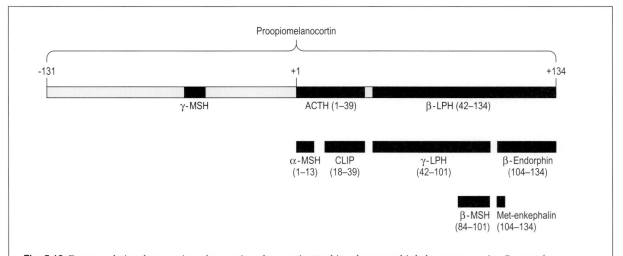

Fig. 5.13 Post-translational processing of pro-opiomelanocorticotrophin releases multiple hormone species. See text for an explanation of abbreviations.

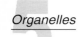

Membrane trafficking

Trafficking between membrane-bounded organelles is mediated by small membrane vesicles, which bud and pinch-off from the source organelle and bind and fuse with the target organelle. In addition to driving membrane invagination in receptor-mediated endocytosis, clathrin (see Chapter 4) has been detected on many intracellular organelles and, thus, presents one mechanism by which vesicles may bud and pinch-off. Passage between organelles is directed along microtubule cytoskeletal elements in an ATP-dependent process (see Chapter 9).

Protein targeting to different cellular destinations

Proteins are targeted to cellular destinations either by specific structural signals within the protein or to a default destination in the absence of a specific signal (Fig. 5.14). A complex series of primary and/or secondary structural protein motifs together with appropriate receptor proteins in the target organelle are likely to play a major role. Compartment-specific retention signals are also important so that protein activities localized to particular compartments are not randomized during interorganelle vesicular transport, e.g. a C-terminal KDEL sequence signals retention of the protein in the ER.

Secretory pathways

The passage of nascent polypeptides from the rough ER and through the Golgi apparatus forms the early stage of the secretory pathway. Some proteins are arrested by specific targeting signals that locate the protein within the secretory pathway, e.g. protein disulphide isomerase to the ER, glycosyl transferases to the Golgi. Those proteins that are not sequestered to locations within the ER and Golgi apparatus, targeted to other organelles, the plasma membrane or secretion are sorted in the trans-Golgi network. Proteins may enter either a **constitutive** or a **regulated** secretory pathway (Fig. 5.15). In the constitutive pathway non-clathrin coated vesicles bud-off continuously from the trans-Golgi network and migrate to the cytoplasmic face of the plasma membrane. Fusion of the vesicle with the plasma membrane releases secreted proteins and introduces transmembrane proteins into the membrane. Extracellular matrix proteins and protein components of the plasma membrane use the constitutive pathway. Non-phosphorylated lysosomal proteins also enter this pathway and it may be that the constitutive pathway is the default pathway for any protein that does not carry a specific address. The constitutive pathway is Ca^{2+}-dependent. The Ca^{2+} may be required for vesicle migration and/or vesile/membrane fusion.

Proteins entering the regulated pathway do so at a much higher concentration and are more actively sequestered by binding to aggregated intralumenal receptors in the trans-Golgi network. For example, proinsulin is sequestered by a 25 kDa receptor protein in the trans-Golgi network. The budding-off of vesicles is driven by the formation of clathrin-coated vesicles, and vesicles are transferred towards the site of release along microtubular fibres. Near the plasma membrane, the vesicles in the regulated pathway interact with a network of F-actin-fodrin filaments, which hold most of the vesicles away from the membrane, preventing fusion. A local rise in $[Ca^{2+}]$, in response to an extracellular stimulus, triggers membrane fusion by promoting depolymerization of the F-actin-fodrin matrix, activation of the F-actin-cleaving enzyme gelosin and the capping of actin filaments. In nerve terminals there is evidence that some secretory vesicles in regulated pathways may be linked directly to voltage-gated Ca^{2+} channels by proteins such as synaptotagmin, such that the vesicle is ideally placed for membrane fusion when the local $[Ca^{2+}]$ rises (see Fig. 8.12).

Targeting of transport vesicles: the SNARE hypothesis

Mechanisms for addressing and sorting transport vesicles remain to be elucidated but are clearly complex. The **SNARE hypothesis** proposes that each transport vesicle possesses one or more specific SNARE proteins (vSNARE) in its membrane and that these bind to cognate SNAREs in the target membrane (tSNARE) (Fig. 5.16), thereby ensuring correct targeting of the vesicle. Possible cellular destinations for any transport vesicle are determined, therefore, by the pattern of localization of SNAREs in subcellular compartments. **Soluble NSF attachment proteins (SNAPs)** are thought to bind to interacting SNAREs (**SNAP receptors**), which, in turn, permit the binding of **NSF proteins** (N-ethylmaleimide-sensitive fusion proteins) to complete the **docking and fusion particle**. How vesicle fusion ensues is unknown but it is thought that ATP hydrolysis by the NSF protein provides the energy for this process.

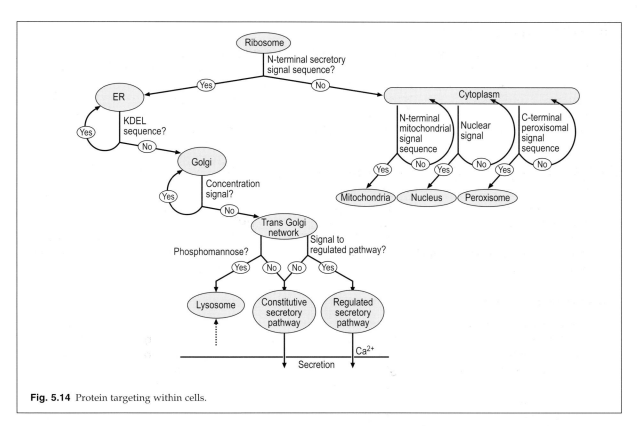

Fig. 5.14 Protein targeting within cells.

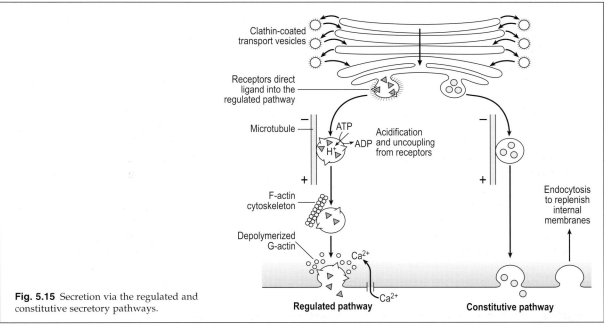

Fig. 5.15 Secretion via the regulated and constitutive secretory pathways.

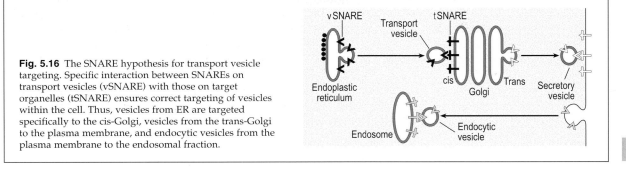

Fig. 5.16 The SNARE hypothesis for transport vesicle targeting. Specific interaction between SNAREs on transport vesicles (vSNARE) with those on target organelles (tSNARE) ensures correct targeting of vesicles within the cell. Thus, vesicles from ER are targeted specifically to the cis-Golgi, vesicles from the trans-Golgi to the plasma membrane, and endocytic vesicles from the plasma membrane to the endosomal fraction.

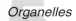

Further reading

Aridor M, Balch W E 1996 Principles of selective transport: coat complexes hold the key. Trends in Cell Biology 6: 315–320

Rothman J E 1994 Mechanisms of intracellular protein transport. Nature 372: 55–83

Schatz G, Dobberstein B 1996 Common principles of protein translocation across membranes. Science 271: 1519–1526

Whiteheart S W, Kubalek E W 1995 SNAPs and NSF: general members of the fusion apparatus. Trends in Cell Biology 5: 64–68

Revision questions

1. How is nuclear DNA packaged in a non-dividing eukaryotic cell?

2. What is the mechanism for communication between cytoplasm and nucleoplasm?

3. Which mitochondrial membrane is important for cellular respiration?

4. Many proteins are imported by mitochondria. Describe the processes by which proteins are thought to be targeted to the intramitochondrial space and the inner and outer membranes.

5. Describe the mechanism by which secretory, lysosomal and membrane proteins are translocated into the endoplasmic reticulum.

6. How is the topology (orientation) of membrane proteins determined?

7. Proteins may be targeted to different cellular destinations by cellular targeting motifs. Where no cellular targeting signal motifs or compartment-specific retention signals are present, where would you expect a membrane protein to be localized?

8. Outline the SNARE hypothesis of transport vesicle targeting.

Answers to revision questions

1. In the non-dividing cell, nuclear DNA is packaged as chromatin (see Fig. 5.2).

2. Nuclear pores allow communication between the nucleoplasm and cytoplasm. Proteins up to ~60 kDa may diffuse freely. Larger molecules may be selectively transported in an ATP-dependent process.

3. The proteins responsible for electron transfer and oxidative phosphorylation are all located on the inner mitochondrial membrane. Unlike the outer membrane, which is relatively permeable, the inner membrane is impermeable to protons and allows the build-up of the electrochemical proton gradient used to drive the synthesis of ATP.

4. Mitochondrial proteins are targeted to the mitochondrion by an N-terminal targeting sequence. This directs vectorial transfer of the protein across the membrane at specific adhesion sites between the outer and inner membranes. Outer membrane proteins are probably located by the presence of stop-transfer sequences within their structure. Once internalized, intermembrane and inner membrane proteins are thought to be targeted back to the inner membrane via a targeting sequence revealed on cleavage of the N-terminal mitochondrial targeting sequence. Insertion of these proteins may be analogous to protein translocation in the ER. Cleavage of the start-transfer sequence releases the translocated protein into the intermembrane space. Inner membrane proteins are probably located by the same mechanism except that their translocation is arrested by the presence of stop-transfer sequences (see Fig. 5.9).

5. Secretory, lysosomal and membrane proteins are targeted to the ER by an N-terminal hydrophobic signal sequence during their synthesis. Synthesis commences in the cytoplasm but is arrested on the ribosome by the binding of a signal recognition particle (SRP) to the signal sequence as it emerges from the ribosome. The arrest of synthesis is released on binding of the SRP to an SRP receptor on the ER. This releases the signal sequence, which interacts with a signal sequence receptor that directs further synthesis through the ER membrane. Ribophorins bind the ribosome to the ER and constitute part of the pore through which the new protein is extruded. Unless a stop-transfer sequence is located in the newly synthesized protein to arrest translocation of a membrane protein, the newly synthesized protein is translocated fully into the lumen of the ER. Where translocation of a membrane protein is arrested, the ribosome must detach from the ER to complete the synthesis of the protein. As soon as they appear in the ER lumen, signal sequences are cleaved from the new protein by signal peptidases (see Fig. 5.7).

6. The topology of most membrane proteins is determined during synthesis by the binding of the signal sequence to the ER membrane. Topology of proteins inserted in the membrane post-translationally is determined by the orientation of the protein by targeting sequences for vectorial transport.

7. The default destination of a membrane protein with no cellular targeting motif or compartment-specific retention signal appears to be the plasma membrane (see Fig. 5.15).

8. The SNARE hypothesis proposes that transport vesicle targeting is achieved through the interaction of vSNAREs on the transport vesicle with cognate tSNAREs on the target membrane.

Cell to cell signalling: chemical signalling and signal transduction across membranes

In multicellular organisms where different functions are carried out by differentiated cells, mechanisms for intercellular communication are required to ensure the efficient integration of cellular activities or **homeostasis**. Signalling between cells may occur directly, through gap junctions between cells (Chapters 8 and 10) or through activation of anchorage-dependent signalling pathways (Chapter 10), or indirectly, via the secretion of extracellular chemical messengers, which cause a response in a target cell when recognized by specific receptors (Fig. 6.1).

Chemical signalling

Intercellular chemical signals may be classified according to their functions into **hormones**, **local mediators** and **neurotransmitters**. A single molecule may fall into more than one of these categories depending on where it is synthesized and released.

- **Hormones** are secreted by specialized cells, usually found in endocrine glands, into the circulation and are carried to target cells where they have their effect (Fig. 6.2A). Endocrine signalling coordinates the activities of distally related tissues (Fig. 6.3).
- **Local mediators** are released by many cells into the extracellular fluid where they produce responses in cells in the same area (Fig. 6.2B). They are often short-lived chemical species and are not found generally in the circulation. Signalling by local mediators is referred to as **paracrine** signalling.
- **Neurotransmitters** are released by nerve cells at nerve terminals into specialized junctions between cells called synapses (Fig. 6.2C). Diffusion of the neurotransmitter across the synapse and binding to receptors on the post-synaptic membrane permits targeted transfer of information between adjacent cells.

Receptors for chemical signals

Definitions

Ligand. A ligand is any small molecule that binds specifically to a receptor site. Ligand binding may produce an activation of a receptor. In this case the ligand is termed an **agonist**. Alternatively, a ligand may combine with a receptor site without causing activation. This type of ligand is termed an **antagonist** because it would oppose the action of an agonist. Agonists that stimulate a receptor but are unable to elicit the maximum cell response possible are termed **partial agonists**.

Receptor. A receptor is a molecule that recognizes specifically a ligand, or family of ligands, and which in response to ligand binding brings about regulation of a cellular process. In the unbound state a receptor is functionally silent. Thus, catecholamine (e.g. adrenaline) binding to a β-adrenergic receptor (β-adrenoceptor) brings about the activation of the enzyme, adenylyl cyclase, and a cascade of signalling events in the cell. Equally, binding to an LDL receptor sets in train the internalization of cholesterol into the cell (see Chapter 4).

Acceptor molecules. Many molecules whose activities are modified by the binding of small chemicals, including drugs, are not strictly receptors under the above definition. If their basic function can be carried out without the interaction of a ligand then they are not, by definition, a receptor. For example, the enzyme dihydrofolate reductase is inhibited by the binding of the drug methotrexate, and is sometimes referred to as the 'methotrexate receptor'. This enzyme operates normally in the absence of methotrexate. Equally, the voltage-gated Na^+ channel opens in response to an electrical event, but can be modulated by the binding of local anaesthetic agents and a variety of neurotoxic molecules and is often referred to as the receptor for these agents. Dihydrofolate reductase and sodium channels both operate in the absence of any signalling molecule. More accurately, these molecules should be referred to as '**acceptor**' molecules because their basic function can occur without the interaction of a ligand.

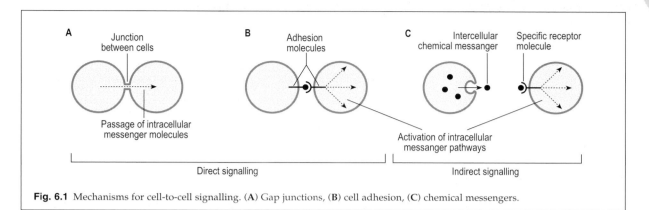

Fig. 6.1 Mechanisms for cell-to-cell signalling. (**A**) Gap junctions, (**B**) cell adhesion, (**C**) chemical messengers.

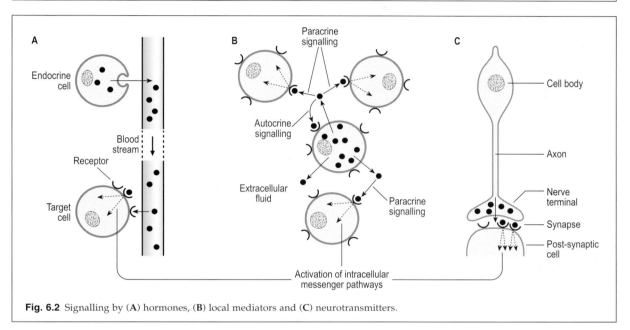

Fig. 6.2 Signalling by (**A**) hormones, (**B**) local mediators and (**C**) neurotransmitters.

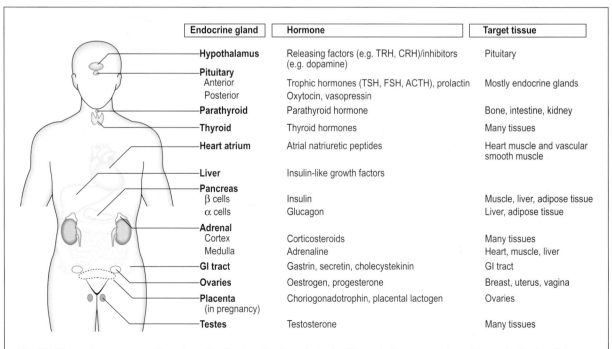

Endocrine gland	Hormone	Target tissue
Hypothalamus	Releasing factors (e.g. TRH, CRH)/inhibitors (e.g. dopamine)	Pituitary
Pituitary Anterior	Trophic hormones (TSH, FSH, ACTH), prolactin	Mostly endocrine glands
Posterior	Oxytocin, vasopressin	
Parathyroid	Parathyroid hormone	Bone, intestine, kidney
Thyroid	Thyroid hormones	Many tissues
Heart atrium	Atrial natriuretic peptides	Heart muscle and vascular smooth muscle
Liver	Insulin-like growth factors	
Pancreas β cells	Insulin	Muscle, liver, adipose tissue
α cells	Glucagon	Liver, adipose tissue
Adrenal Cortex	Corticosteroids	Many tissues
Medulla	Adrenaline	Heart, muscle, liver
GI tract	Gastrin, secretin, cholecystekinin	GI tract
Ovaries	Oestrogen, progesterone	Breast, uterus, vagina
Placenta (in pregnancy)	Choriogonadotrophin, placental lactogen	Ovaries
Testes	Testosterone	Many tissues

Fig. 6.3 The endocrine system. Location of endocrine glands in the body. The main hormones released by each gland and their tissue targets are shown.

Specificity of response

For a cell to respond to any chemical messenger it must produce specific receptor proteins that recognize and produce a response to the signalling molecule. If the signalling molecule is hydrophilic the signal recognition site of the receptor must be present on the extracellular face of the cell surface. Interaction of the signalling molecule with its specific receptor must then result in the activation of a cellular process. If the signalling molecule is hydrophobic the signal will be able to gain access to the cell through the lipid bilayer by diffusion but an intracellular receptor is still required to transduce the signal into a cellular response. The presence or absence of a specific receptor in a cell governs the responsiveness of that cell to any signalling molecule.

Classification of receptors

Receptors are classified according to the specific physiological signalling molecule (agonist) that they recognize, e.g. acetylcholine receptors (AChR). Further subclassification is made on the basis of their ability to be selectively activated by agonist molecules (Tables 6.1 and 6.2). Subclassification is also often made on the basis of the affinity (a measure of tightness of binding) of a series of antagonists (Tables 6.1 and 6.2).

Properties of receptor binding sites

Analogies can be drawn between receptor binding sites and the active sites and regulatory sites of enzymes.

Similarities

- Binding at both receptor sites and enzyme sites is specific.
- The specificity of binding is governed by the shape of the binding cleft in the receptor or enzyme site.
- The specificity of binding confers specificity to the regulation of processes in which receptors are involved or the specificity for substrate of an enzyme.
- Binding to both receptors and enzymes is usually reversible.
- Ligand binding to receptor and regulator binding to enzyme allosteric sites both induce a conformational change and a change in the activity of the molecule (substrate molecules may also 'induce a fit').
- There is no chemical modification of ligand in receptor binding sites or enzyme regulatory sites.

Differences

- The affinity of ligand binding at receptor sites is generally higher than the binding of substrates and regulators to enzyme sites. The concentration of ligand that half fills all available receptor sites (the dissociation constant, K_D) is generally in the nanomolar (10^{-9} M) to micromolar (10^{-6} M) concentration range. Often the concentration of substrate that half fills available enzyme active sites (Michaelis constant, K_M) is in the micromolar (10^{-6} M) to millimolar (10^{-3} M) concentration range.
- The ligand bound to a receptor site is not modified chemically whereas substrate bound in an enzyme active site is modified in a chemical reaction catalysed by the active site.

Signal transduction

Some hydrophobic signalling molecules are able to cross the plasma membrane freely and interact with intracellular receptors to bring about changes in cellular activity (e.g. steroid and thyroid hormones). Most signalling molecules are hydrophilic and are unable to cross the plasma membrane. To exert their effect, hydrophilic signalling molecules must interact with specific receptor proteins at the cell surface.

Common mechanisms used to transduce an extracellular signal into an intracellular event include:

1. membrane-bound receptors with integral ion channels
2. membrane-bound receptors with integral enzyme activity
3. membrane-bound receptors that couple to effectors through transducing proteins
4. intracellular receptors.

Receptor type Receptor Subtype		Muscarinic			Nicotinic
		M₁	M₂	M₃	
Agonists	Acetylcholine	+++	+++	+++	+++
	Carbamylcholine	++	++	++	+++
	Muscarine	+++	+++	+++	−
	Nicotine	−	−	−	+++
Antagonists	Atropine	+++	+++	+++	−
	Pirenzepine	+++	+	+	−
	Gallamine	+	+++	+	+++
	Hexahydrosiladiphenidol	++	+	+++	−

Table 6.1 Classification of acetylcholine receptor types and subtypes by their specificity for agonists and antagonists

		Subtype			
		α₁	α₂	β₁	β₂
Agonists	Noradrenaline	+++	+++	++	+
	Adrenaline	++	++	++++	+++
	Isoprenaline	−	−	+++	+++
	Phenylephrine	++	−	−	−
	Clonidine	−	+++	−	−
	Methyl noradrenaline	+	+++	−	−
	Salbutamol	−	−	+	+++
	Dobutamine	−	−	+++	+
Antagonists	Phentolamine	+++	+++	−	−
	Yohimbine	+	+++	−	−
	Prazosin	+++	+	−	−
	Propranolol	−	−	+++	+++
	Atenolol	−	−	+++	+
	Butoxamine	−	−	+	+++

Table 6.2 Classification of adrenoceptor subtypes by their specificity for agonists and antagonists

Membrane-bound receptors with integral ion channels: ligand-gated ion channels

Agonist binding to ligand-gated ion channels results in a change in conformation and opening of a gated channel, which permits the flow of ions down an electrochemical gradient. This transduces the chemical signal into an electrical event at the plasma membrane.

Several receptors of this type belong to the 'classical' ligand-gated ion channel family that have similar pentameric structures (Table 6.3, Fig. 6.4). In addition to the 'classical' ligand-gated ion channels in the plasma membrane, other structurally distinct ligand-gated ion channel families can also be present in cells (Table 6.3, Fig. 6.4). In addition, several agonists that act normally through G-protein-coupled receptors, e.g. adrenaline, angiotensin II and histamine, open plasma membrane ion channels. The nature of these receptor-operated channels remains to be determined. In some cases this channel activity may represent G-protein activation of normally voltage-operated channels but the possibility of novel distinct ligand-gated ion channels cannot be ruled out.

Ligand-gated ion channels may also be present on intracellular membranes to respond to intracellular signals. For example, inositol 1,4,5-trisphosphate (InsP$_3$) interaction with InsP$_3$ receptors in the endoplasmic reticulum opens a Ca^{2+} channel that releases stored Ca^{2+} into the cytoplasm (see Chapter 7). Ca^{2+} itself may also stimulate opening of these channels. A second related channel, the ryanodine-sensitive calcium channel (ryanodine receptor, RyR) opens normally in response to raised [Ca^{2+}]$_i$ but may also be activated by a novel NAD$^+$-derived second messenger, cyclic ADP-ribose.

Myasthenia gravis

Muscle weakness in patients with the autoimmune condition myasthenia gravis is due to the presence of antibodies directed against nicotinic acetylcholine receptors. Binding of antibodies induces an increased rate of receptor degradation and complement-dependent lysis of muscle fibres.

Membrane-bound receptors with integral enzyme activity

Agonist binding to the extracellular domain of these receptors causes a conformational change that activates an intrinsic enzyme activity contained within the cytoplasmic domain of the receptor (Fig. 6.5). In this way extracellular messages are transduced either into intracellular chemical messages, **second messenger molecules** (e.g. cyclic GMP), or via the modification of activities of cytoplasmic proteins by covalent phosphorylation or dephosphorylation (Table 6.4). Dimerization of these single transmembrane-spanning polypeptide receptors is probably required for activity of all receptors in this group.

Atrial natriuretic peptide (ANP) signals vasorelaxation through an enzyme-linked receptor

ANP released from the atrium in response to atrial stretch, e.g. in response to volume expansion or cardiac failure, acts on vascular smooth muscle to stimulate the production of the intracellular messenger cyclic GMP and vasorelaxation, thus causing a reduction in blood pressure.

Tyrosine kinase-linked receptors

Signalling via tyrosine kinase-linked receptors involves covalent modification of the receptor itself. Binding of hormone to extracellular binding sites activates a protein tyrosine kinase activity in the cytoplasmic domain of the receptor protein, which autophosphorylates (catalyses the transfer of a phosphate group from ATP onto its own structure) tyrosine residues on the cytoplasmic domain of the receptor. Phosphorylated receptor tyrosine residues are recognized either by transducing proteins, e.g. insulin receptor substrate-1 (IRS-1), or directly by enzymes containing phosphotyrosine recognition sites, **Src homology-2 (SH2)** domains (Fig. 6.6). On association with receptor or transducing protein, effector enzymes become activated allosterically, or possibly by tyrosine phosphorylation by the receptor kinase, thus transducing the message into an intracellular chemical event.

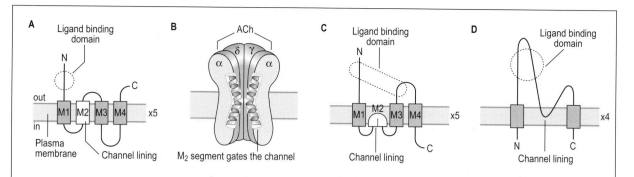

Fig. 6.4 Structure of ligand-gated ion channels. (**A**) Membrane topography of subunits of the 'classic' ligand-gated ion channel family. (**B**) Cross-sectional view of a pentameric nicotinic acetylcholine receptor. Charged residues in the mouth of the channel determine the cation selectivity of the channel. (**C**) Members of the glutamate receptor family have a slightly different membrane topography. (**D**) Membrane topography of the P_{2X} purinergic receptor (note the similarity to the structure of the inward rectifier K^+ channel family, see Chapter 8).

Receptor	Subunit structure	Ligand	Ligand binding subunit	Channel
Nicotinic acetylcholine (nAChR)	$\alpha_2\beta\epsilon\delta$ (adult) $\alpha_2\beta\gamma\delta$ (fetal)	Acetylcholine	α	Na^+ predominantly, and K^+ ions (excitatory)
Glycine	$\alpha_3\beta_2$	Glycine	α	Cl^- (inhibitory)
GABA_A	5 subunits e.g. $\alpha_2\beta_2\gamma$	GABA*	α	Cl^- (inhibitory)
Glutamate (e.g. NMDA, AMPA and kainate receptors)	5 subunits	Glutamate/ aspartate		Ca^{2+} (excitatory)

Table 6.3 Examples of 'classical' ligand-gated ion channels. AMPA, α-amino-3-hydroxy-5-methyl-4-isoxazoleproprionate; NMDA, N-methyl-D-aspartate; GABA, γ-amino butyric acid. *Benzodiazepine binding to the β subunit potentiates the action of GABA

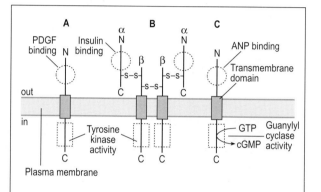

Fig. 6.5 Membrane-bound receptors with integral enzyme activity. (**A**) The platelet-derived growth factor (PDGF) receptor and (**B**) insulin receptor both possess integral tyrosine kinase domains while (**C**) the atrial natriuretic peptide (ANP) receptor possesses an integral guanylyl cyclase domain. Monomeric receptors dimerize on activation.

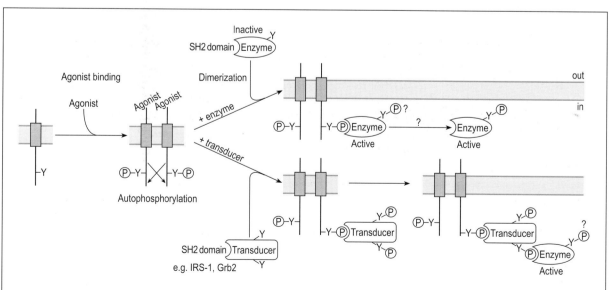

Fig. 6.6 Signal transduction by tyrosine-kinase-linked receptors. Receptor autophosphorylation is stimulated in response to agonist binding. Effector enzymes interact with the autophosphorylated receptor either directly or indirectly via a transducing protein e.g. IRS-1, Grb2. Interactions with phosphotyrosine residues (Y-P) contained within short specific amino acid sequences is mediated by SH2 domains in the transducer and effector proteins.

Membrane-bound receptors with no integral enzyme or channel activity: seven transmembrane domain receptors

Seven transmembrane domain receptors couple to effector molecules via a transducing molecule, a **GTP-binding regulatory protein (G-protein)**. This family of receptors is also known as the **G-protein-coupled receptor** family. Effectors may be enzymes or ion channels. For example, in cardiac pacemaker cells, acetylcholine binding to M_2 muscarinic acetylcholine receptors inhibits adenylyl cyclase activity and stimulates K^+ channel opening via a G-protein, G_i.

A wide variety of extracellular signalling molecules use specific seven transmembrane domain receptors and, thus, there is an extensive superfamily of proteins with this common structure (Fig. 6.7). Examples include: muscarinic acetylcholine receptors (mAChR stimulated by muscarine), adrenoceptors (for adrenaline and noradrenaline), dopamine receptors, 5-hydroxytryptamine (5-HT) receptors, opioid receptors, peptide receptors (e.g. substance P, angiotensin) purine (P_{2Y}) receptors (e.g. ATP), light receptors (rhodopsin), smell and taste receptors and many others. Often many different types of receptor exist for a particular agonist, each with its own pharmacology (e.g. Tables 6.1 and 6.2).

Intracellular receptors

Hydrophobic ligands, such as the steroid hormones, cortisol, oestrogen and testosterone and the thyroid hormones T_3 and T_4, penetrate the plasma membrane and bind to monomeric receptors in the cytoplasm or nucleus. In the resting state these receptors are stabilized by association with heat shock or chaperone proteins. The activated receptor dissociates from the chaperone protein and translocates to the nucleus where it binds to control regions in the DNA defined by specific sequences, thereby regulating gene expression. DNA binding occurs through a region of conserved amino acid sequence known as a 'zinc finger' that is present in many proteins known to regulate DNA transcription (Fig. 6.8). Compared with receptors that activate channels or enzymes (reviewed above), the effects of intracellular receptor activation are relatively slow in onset because transcription and translation are required.

Transducing proteins

Many membrane receptors employ intermediary proteins to transduce the events of receptor activation to effector molecules in the cell, e.g. IRS-1 and IRS-2 (see above) and GTP-binding regulatory proteins.

Heteromeric GTP-binding regulatory proteins (G-proteins)

The heteromeric G-proteins are a large family of proteins that transduce the signal from seven transmembrane domain (G-protein-coupled) receptors to a variety of effector molecules (Table 6.5). Each G-protein has a common heterotrimeric structure of three distinct subunits: alpha (α) bound to GDP, beta (β) and gamma (γ) (Fig. 6.9). Receptor activation induces a conformational change in the G-protein. This change in structure causes the release of GDP. GTP binds in its place and the α-GTP and $\beta\gamma$ complex both dissociate from the receptor and go on to interact with, and activate or inhibit, specific effector molecules. A slow integral GTPase activity in the α subunit hydrolyses GTP and returns the α subunit to its inactive conformation and α-GDP$\beta\gamma$ heterotrimers reform. Thus, the duration of the intracellular signal is controlled by rate of GTP hydrolysis by the α subunit. In this way G-proteins act as a molecular **switch** (GDP/GTP exchange) to activate intracellular effector molecules but also as a **timer** (GTP hydrolysis) to ensure that the cellular activation is transient and occurs only while the extracellular signalling molecule is present at the cell surface.

G-protein diversity

G-protein coupling is a widely used mechanism with many permutations. At least 20 different α, five β and eight γ subunits have been identified by molecular biological analysis. Different combinations of these can couple over 500 different receptors to at least 10 enzyme or ion channel effector molecules (examples given in Table 6.5). Several subfamilies of α subunits have been identified and the nature of a G-protein is defined by the α subunit present. These include G_s (stimulates adenylyl cyclase), G_i (inhibits adenylyl cyclase), G_q, (stimulates phospholipase C, see Chapter 7) and G_t (transducin in retinal rod cells which transduces the detection of light into enzyme activation, see Chapter 8).

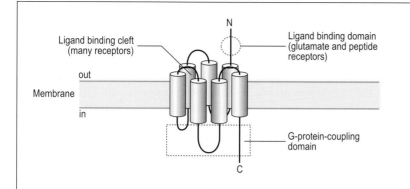

Fig. 6.7 Structure of seven transmembrane domain, G-protein-coupled receptors. Agonist binding, usually in a cleft formed by the seven transmembrane domains, induces a conformational change in the internal loops of the receptor. This is transmitted to interacting G-proteins which transduce the signal to effector molecules (Table 6.5).

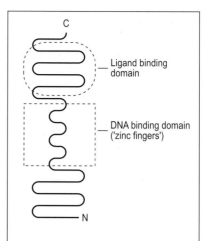

Fig. 6.8 Structure of intracellular receptors.

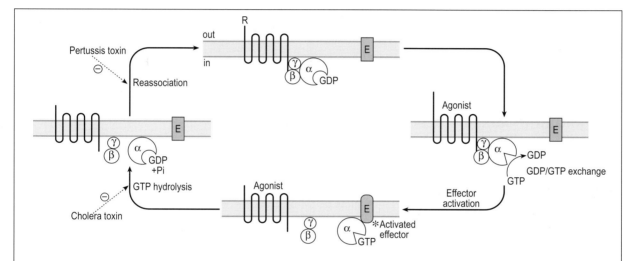

Fig. 6.9 Model for G-protein mediated signal transduction from G-protein-coupled receptors to effector proteins. Transduction may be mediated by free α GTP subunits or by free βγ subunit complex (Table 6.5). E, effector protein; R, receptor; * indicates activation. Two bacterial toxins, **cholera toxin** from the bacterium *Vibrio cholerae* and **pertussis toxin** from the **whooping cough** bacterium *Bordetella pertussis*, have been most useful in distinguishing G-protein coupling mechanisms in many signalling pathways. Both toxins result in the enzymatic transfer of an ADP-ribosyl group from NAD+ to an arginine residue in the G-protein α subunit. Cholera toxin modifies $G_s\alpha$ rendering the GTPase activity inactive and, thereby, the G-protein constitutively active. By contrast, ADP-ribosylation of $G_i\alpha$ by pertussis toxin prevents association of the $G_i\alpha\beta\gamma$ complex with its receptor and, thereby, prevents agonist-induced dissociation of the G_i complex. This produces an inhibition of the G_i inhibitory pathway in the cell. Steps inhibited by cholera toxin (G_s) and pertussis toxin (G_i, G_0) are indicated.

Effector enzyme activity	Ligand	Receptor
Tyrosine kinase	Epidermal growth factor (EGF)	EGF receptor
	Insulin	Insulin receptor
	Platelet-derived growth factor (PDGF)	PDGF receptor
Phosphoprotein phosphatase	Antigen	Leucocyte common antigen (CD45)
	Adhesion molecules	Leucocyte common antigen related protein (LAR)
Guanylyl cyclase	Atrial natriuretic peptide (ANP)	ANP receptor

Table 6.4 Enzyme-linked receptors

G-protein subunit	Effector(s)
$G_s\alpha$-GTP	↑ adenylyl cyclase
	↑ Ca²⁺ channels
βγ (from $G_i\alpha\beta\gamma$)	↓ adenylyl cyclase
βγ (from cardiac muscarinic receptor activation)	↑ K⁺ channel
$G_{i2}\alpha$-GTP	↓ adenylyl cyclase
$G_t\alpha$-GTP (transducin)	↑ cGMP phosphodiesterase
$G_q\alpha$-GTP	↑ PtdInsP₂-PLC
$G_{oA}\alpha$-GTP	↓ Ca²⁺ channels

Table 6.5 Some G-proteins and their effectors. Note: signal transduction via G-proteins may be excitatory or inhibitory. PLC, phospholipase C; PtdInsP₂, phosphatidylinositol 4,5-bisphosphate

Monomeric G-proteins

Initially identified as products of viral oncogenes (cancer-inducing genes), a second family of monomeric GTP-binding regulatory proteins has been characterized. A member of this family, Ras, is responsible for producing tumours of connective tissue (sarcomas). In normal cells these G-proteins participate in signalling pathways involved in the transmission of signals from tyrosine kinase-linked receptors in pathways concerned with the regulation of cell growth and differentiation. However, unlike the trimeric G-proteins, the Ras proteins do not interact directly with the membrane receptor (Fig. 6.10). High concentrations of Ras proteins are often found in proliferating and immature cells.

The Ras proteins, like the heterotrimeric G-protein α subunits, bind GDP in the inactive state and GTP when activated. In this case, nucleotide exchange is stimulated by **guanine-nucleotide releasing proteins (GNRPs)**, such as Grb2 and Sos (Fig. 6.10). As with the trimeric G-proteins, the Ras protein is inactivated on slow hydrolysis of GTP. This can be increased over 100-fold by the interaction of **GTPase-activating proteins (GAP)**.

Ras couples tyrosine kinase receptor signalling to cell growth and differentiation. Other members of the Ras family couple tyrosine kinase receptor signalling to the cytoskeleton (Rho), vesicle transport (Rab, ARF) and nuclear protein import (Ran1).

Point mutations in *ras* are oncogenic

Analysis of the amino acid sequence of Ras proteins in viral and human cancers reveals that single point mutations can be sufficient to transform these genes into oncogenes (see Chapter 13). In the oncogenic form, GTPase activity is even slower than normal.

SH2 and SH3 domains in adapter proteins

SH2 and SH3 homology domains, initially identified in the *src* oncogene product, are common in signalling pathway proteins and permit protein–protein association. SH2 domains recognize phosphotyrosine residues within specific short amino acid sequences and SH3 domains recognize amino acid sequences rich in proline residues. Some proteins are composed almost entirely of SH2 and SH3 domains, e.g. Grb2, and these act as docking proteins or adapters between cellular proteins when tyrosine kinase activity has been stimulated.

Amplification of extracellular signals

The concentration of many extracellular signalling molecules is very low (10^{-12}–10^{-6} M). In each of the above receptor-mediated mechanisms there is the possibility of molecular amplification. For example, by stimulating the activity of an enzyme, the binding of a chemical signal molecule to a single receptor can cause the modification of hundreds or thousands of substrate molecules. A cascade of such catalytic events can produce further amplification (Fig. 6.11).

Cellular activation and inhibition

Responses to receptor activation can lead to cellular activation or inhibition depending on the receptor. For example:

- In cardiac pacemaker cells, noradrenaline acting on β_1-adrenoceptors produces an increased heart rate, while acetylcholine acting on M_2 muscarinic receptors produces a slowing of the heart rate.
- In smooth muscle, acetylcholine acting on M_3 muscarinic receptors stimulates contraction, while adrenaline acting on β_2-adrenoceptors inhibits contraction.
- In hepatocytes, insulin stimulates the synthesis of glycogen from glucose and inhibits glycogen breakdown while glucagon inhibits glycogen synthesis and stimulates glycogen breakdown.

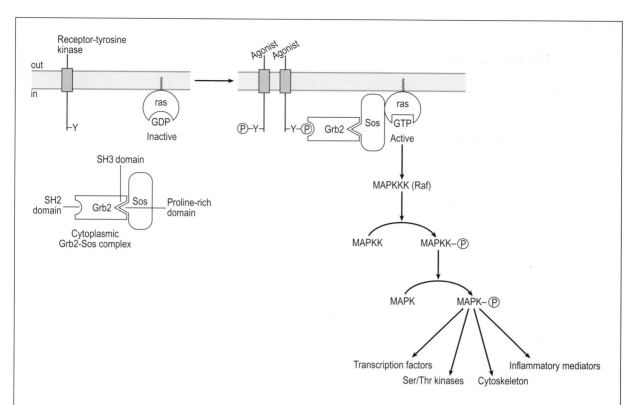

Fig. 6.10 Role of Ras in coupling receptor tyrosine kinase activation to the activation of cytoplasmic mitogen-activated protein kinase (MAPK) via sequential activation of raf (mitogen-activated protein kinase kinase kinase, MAPKKK) and mitogen-activated protein kinase kinase (MAPKK or MEK). Grb2 binding to phosphotyrosine residues on the autophosphorylated receptor localize bound Sos to the membrane, where it induces GDP dissociation from Ras and, hence, GTP binding and activation.

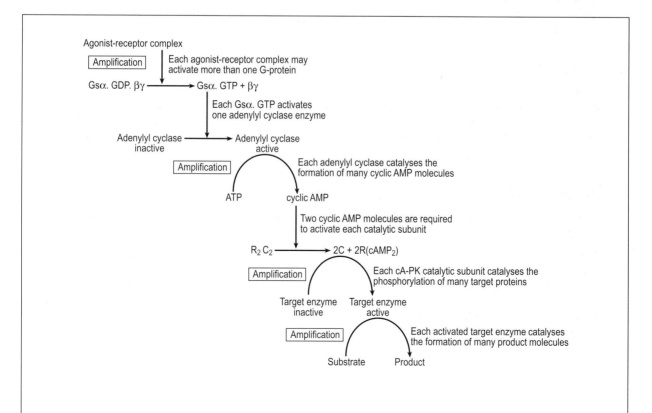

Fig. 6.11 Amplification of extracellular signals in the adenylyl cyclase → cyclic AMP → cyclic AMP-dependent protein kinase signalling pathway.

Further reading

Aidley D J, Stanfield P R 1996 Ion channels: molecules in action. Cambridge University Press, Cambridge

Barritt G J 1992 Communication within animal cells. Oxford University Press, Oxford

Bourne H R, Sanders D A, McCormick F 1991 The GTPase superfamily: conserved structure and molecular mechanism. Nature 349: 117–127

Mangelsdorf D J, Thummel C, Beato M, et al. 1995 The nuclear receptor superfamily – the 2nd decade. Cell 83: 835–839

Neer E J 1995 Heterotrimeric G-proteins – organizers of transmembrane signals. Cell 80: 249–257

Rang H P, Dale M M 1995 Pharmacology, 3rd edn. Churchill Livingstone, Edinburgh

Revision questions

1. Define the term 'ligand'.

2. Define the term 'receptor'.

3. How are receptor subtypes defined pharmacologically?

4. Describe the mechanisms by which the following receptors can transduce the message carried by an extracellular signalling molecule into an intracellular event: (a) the nicotinic acetylcholine receptor, (b) muscarinic acetylcholine receptors, (c) the insulin receptor, (d) the atrial natriuretic peptide receptor, (e) steroid hormone receptors.

5. Draw a diagram to illustrate the activation of G-proteins by agonist-stimulated G-protein-coupled receptors.

6. Cholera toxin and pertussis toxin both modify guanine-nucleotide binding proteins by ADP-ribosylation of an α subunit. One toxin results in activation of a G-protein while the other is inhibitory. Explain how the action of both toxins can result in elevated levels of cyclic AMP.

7. What is the function of *src* homology domains 2 and 3 in cellular signalling pathways?

Answers to revision questions

1. A ligand is any small molecule that binds specifically to a receptor site.

2. A receptor is a molecule that recognizes specifically a ligand, or family of ligands, and which in response to ligand binding brings about regulation of a cellular process.

3. Receptors are classified according to the specific physiological signalling molecule (agonist) that they recognize. Selectivity for agonists and antagonists is then used to subclassify receptors further (c.f. Tables 6.1 and 6.2).

4. (a) ligand-gated cation channel activation and membrane depolarization
   (b) G-protein dissociation and activation of effector enzymes and channels
   (c) activation of integral receptor-tyrosine kinase activity, autophosphorylation followed by interaction with and activation of effector enzymes
   (d) activation of guanylyl cyclase to produce the second messenger cyclic GMP which goes on to activate protein kinase G
   (e) activated steroid hormone receptors act directly as transactivating factors in gene transcription.

5. c.f. Fig. 6.9.

6. Cholera toxin results in constitutive activity of the G_s G-protein and, thus, increased stimulation of adenylyl cyclase. By preventing the association of G_i G-protein with inhibitory receptors, the inhibitory influence of G_i on adenylyl cyclase activity is removed by pertussis toxin, resulting in a greater response to G_s activation.

7. SH2 domains recognize phosphotyrosine residues within short specific amino acid sequences while SH3 domains recognize short proline-rich sequences. Both domains provide a mechanism for targeting intracellular protein interactions.

Signal transduction: intracellular signalling pathways

Activation of some receptors results in the direct transduction of the signal into an intracellular response. For example, conformational changes in ligand-gated ion channels in response to agonist binding result in opening of an ion channel and a resultant change in membrane potential. Similarly, activated thyroid hormone receptors in the nucleus transduce the message at the level of gene expression by binding directly to sites in the DNA. The response to activation of many receptors is less direct. In these cases, cascades of intracellular cell signalling events are initiated via cell signalling pathways consisting of transducing proteins, intracellular messenger molecules and effector enzymes.

Second messengers

In many instances the response to receptor activation is the activation of an enzyme effector, which produces a small intracellular messenger molecule or '**second messenger**'. So that intracellular signalling occurs only during receptor activation, second messengers must:

- be maintained at low concentration in the resting cell
- be produced only in response to activation of specific receptors
- be produced in proportion to the size of the extracellular signal
- produce a cellular response in proportion to the change in concentration of the second messenger
- be degraded rapidly to ensure transiency in signalling pathways.

Cyclic nucleotides

Cyclic adenosine 3′,5′-monophosphate (cyclic AMP, cAMP) is produced by an integral plasma membrane enzyme, **adenylyl cyclase**, which converts ATP to cyclic AMP and pyrophosphate (Fig. 7.1). Adenylyl cyclase is activated by receptors that couple through G_s, e.g. β-adrenoceptors (adrenaline/noradrenaline), dopaminergic D_1, glucagon and growth hormone receptors, while receptors coupling through G_i produce an inhibitory response, e.g. $α_2$-adrenoceptors and dopaminergic D_2 receptors. Note that a given agonist many be excitatory or inhibitory depending on the receptor expressed by a cell. The second messenger, cyclic AMP, transmits the signal through the cell by diffusion to cyclic AMP-dependent protein kinase (PKA or cA-PK), which is then activated to phosphorylate a variety of target proteins within the cell to produce either an activation or inhibition of their activity (e.g. Fig. 7.2).

Activation of adenylyl cyclase to produce cyclic AMP is important in many cellular responses, including increasing hepatic gluconeogenesis and glycogenolysis while inhibiting glycogen synthesis (Fig. 7.2), increasing lipolysis in adipose tissue, producing positive inotropic (force) and chronotropic (rate) responses in the heart and relaxation in smooth muscle. Note, in olfactory cells, rather than act via cA-PK, cyclic AMP acts directly to open cyclic AMP-gated ion channels.

Cyclic AMP is rapidly hydrolysed by cellular cyclic AMP phosphodiesterases, which ensure a rapid return to basal levels once the extracellular stimulus is removed from the cell (Fig. 7.1). Caffeine and theophylline both inhibit cyclic AMP phosphodiesterase and, therefore, act in synergy with adenylyl cyclase activation to produce a larger cyclic AMP response for a given extracellular signal.

Cyclic guanosine 3′,5′-monophosphate (cyclic GMP) (Fig. 7.3A) is produced from GTP by **guanylyl cyclases**, which may be activated either as integral enzyme domains within receptors, e.g. atrial natriuretic peptide (ANP) receptor (see Chapter 6), or free guanylyl cyclase enzymes in the cytoplasm, e.g. activated by **nitric oxide** (NO). Like cyclic AMP, cyclic GMP goes on to activate a specific protein kinase (**protein kinase G**) and is hydrolysed rapidly by cyclic GMP phosphodiesterase to guanosine-5′-monophosphate (5′-GMP). Cyclic GMP is important in relaxation of smooth muscle cells in response to ANP and NO (otherwise known as **endothelium-derived relaxing factor, EDRF**) (Fig. 7.3B). It is noteworthy that a reduction in cyclic GMP levels signals detection of light in retinal cells (see Fig. 8.17).

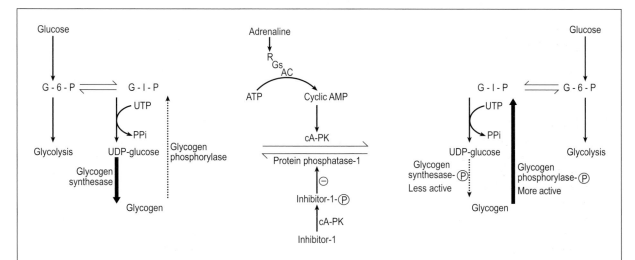

Fig. 7.1 Synthesis and breakdown of cyclic AMP.

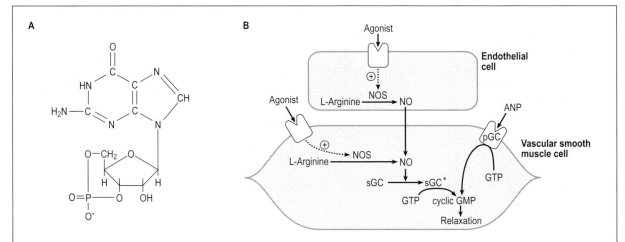

Fig. 7.2 Concerted action of cyclic AMP-dependent protein kinase (cA-PK) in the mobilization of glucose stores. cA-PK phosphorylates phosphorylase kinase (not shown) which phosphorylates and activates glycogen phosphorylase (GP) and, hence, glycogen breakdown. Direct phosphorylation of glycogen synthetase (GS) by cA-PK reduces the activity of GS and hence glycogen synthesis. In addition, cA-PK mediated phosphorylation of protein phosphatase inhibitor-1 reduces the dephosphorylation of enzymes and maintains glycogen breakdown while cyclic AMP levels remain elevated. R, receptor; AC, adenylyl cyclase; G-1-P, glucose-1-phosphate; G-6-P, glucose-6-phosphate.

Fig. 7.3 (**A**) Structure of guanosine 3′,5′-monophosphate (cyclic GMP). (**B**) Relaxation in vascular smooth muscle in response to cyclic GMP. Cyclic GMP may be synthesized by direct activation of particulate (receptor-coupled) guanylyl cyclase (pGC), e.g. by ANP, or by stimulation of soluble guanylyl cyclase (sGC) by nitric oxide (NO). NO may be produced in adjacent endothelial cells by agonist or shear-activation of NO synthase (NOS) or within the vascular smooth muscle cell itself in response to agonist activation.

Phospholipid-derived second messengers

Second messengers derived from phosphatidylinositol 4,5-bisphosphate

A widely used substrate for the generation of second messengers is the minor phospholipid **phosphatidylinositol 4,5-bisphosphate** (PtdInsP$_2$) (Fig. 7.4). Activation of PtdInsP$_2$ phosphodiesterase (**phospholipase C**, PLC) releases the phospholipid head group, **inositol 1,4,5-trisphosphate** (InsP$_3$) leaving **diacylglycerol** (DAG) in the membrane (Fig. 7.4). Both of these hydrolysis products are second messengers (Fig. 7.5).

Inositol 1,4,5-trisphosphate

Inositol 1,4,5-trisphosphate is hydrophilic and diffuses in the cytoplasm to the endo(sarco)plasmic reticulum (ER) where it activates specific InsP$_3$ receptors. These receptors act as second messenger-gated Ca^{2+} channels and cause the release of intracellular Ca^{2+} stores from the lumen of the ER into the cytoplasm. The released Ca^{2+} then acts as a further second messenger by activating Ca^{2+}-dependent processes within the cell. InsP$_3$ may be acted upon by InsP$_3$ 5-phosphatase to produce inositol 1,4-bisphosphate, which is inactive at InsP$_3$ receptors, leading to termination of the signal. Alternatively, in some cells InsP$_3$ may be acted on by InsP$_3$ kinase to produce inositol 1,3,4,5-tetrakisphosphate (InsP$_4$), which represents a further putative second messenger. InsP$_4$ may be involved in raising intracellular Ca^{2+} concentrations, either by facilitating the movement of Ca^{2+} between intracellular vesicular stores or by stimulating store refilling from the extracellular medium (Fig. 7.5). InsP$_4$ is degraded to inositol 1,3,4-trisphosphate, which does not stimulate the InsP$_3$ receptor or InsP$_4$-sensitive mechanisms.

Diacylglycerol

DAG released from PtdInsP$_2$ acts, within the membrane, as an activator of the protein kinase C (PKC) family of enzymes (Fig. 7.5) by reducing the concentration-dependence on [Ca^{2+}]$_i$ (so that it becomes active at lower [Ca^{2+}]$_i$). Since Ca^{2+} also activates this enzyme, the two arms of the signalling pathway from PtdInsP$_2$ act in synergy. Ca^{2+} also stimulates the translocation of PKC from the cytoplasm to the plasma membrane. DAG is removed either by conversion to monoacylglycerol or the action of DAG kinase to form phosphatidic acid (Fig. 7.5).

Range of receptors that activate phosphoinositide hydrolysis

A large number of G-protein-coupled receptors can activate the PtdInsP$_2$ pathway (e.g. muscarinic M$_1$ and M$_3$ (acetylcholine) receptors, H$_1$ (histamine) receptors, α_1-adrenoceptors (noradrenaline), 5-HT$_2$ (serotonin) receptors).

Signalling via the phosphoinositide pathway is important for many cellular responses, including contraction in vascular, gastrointestinal tract and airways smooth muscle, platelet aggregation and mast cell degranulation.

Lithium, phosphoinositide metabolism and the treatment of manic depression

Lithium is used clinically to stabilize mood in the treatment of bipolar manic depression and acute mania. A well-characterized biochemical action of lithium is to inhibit the last step in the dephosphorylation of phosphoinositides to free inositol. It is possible, therefore, that the action of lithium in manic patients is to reduce levels of inositol phospholipids important in signal transduction in the brain. A definite therapeutic role cannot be assigned, however, as this ion also depresses cyclic AMP production and Na$^+$–K$^+$-ATPase activity as well as having effects on neurotransmitter turnover and release.

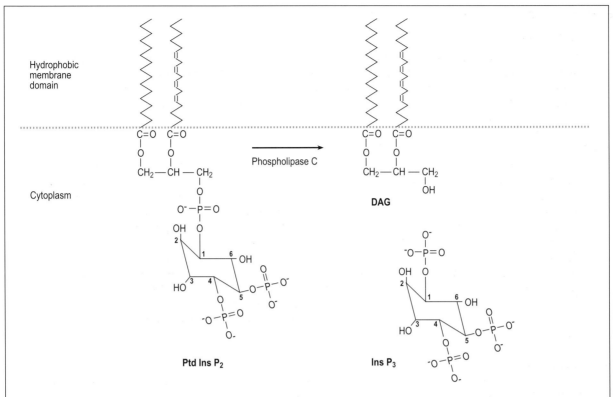

Fig. 7.4 Hydrolysis of phosphatidylinositol 4,5-bisphosphate (PtdInsP$_2$) produces two second messengers, inositol 1,4,5-trisphosphate (InsP$_3$) and 1,2-diacylglycerol (DAG).

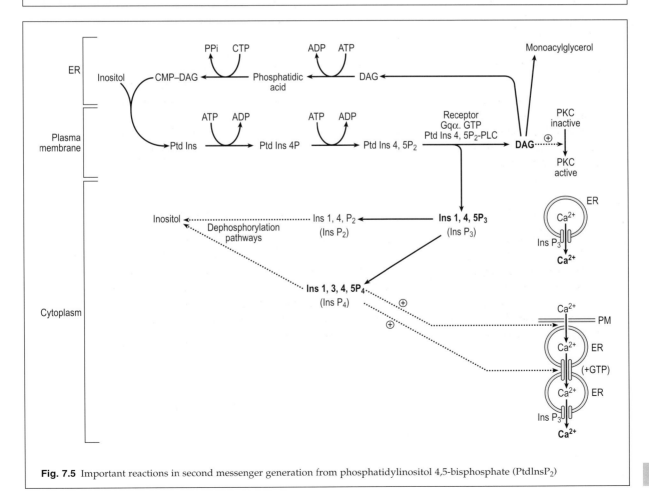

Fig. 7.5 Important reactions in second messenger generation from phosphatidylinositol 4,5-bisphosphate (PtdInsP$_2$)

Second messengers from other phospholipids

In some cells, production of DAG in response to cell activation is prolonged and greater than could be provided by $PtdInsP_2$ breakdown alone. The pathways involved are complex, involving the hydrolysis of phosphatidylcholine and other non-inositol phospholipids by additional phospholipases. The relative contribution of different pathways to the production of DAG varies not only between cell types but also depends on the particular activating agonist.

Local chemical mediators arising from phospholipid metabolism

Further oxidative metabolism of arachidonic acid, released in response to cell stimulation, along the eicosanoid pathways, can result in the production of leukotrienes, prostaglandins and thromboxanes (the eicosanoids) (Fig. 7.6, Table 7.1). These molecules diffuse from the initiating cell and are known to act as local chemical messengers, binding to specific receptors in adjacent cells. In this way a tissue may give a concerted response even when all cells were not activated by the primary messenger and the response in the initiating cell may also be amplified. This latter action is called an autocoid effect.

The non-steroidal anti-inflammatory drugs

The anti-inflammatory action of **non-steroidal anti-inflammatory drugs (NSAIDs)**, such as aspirin (acetyl salicylate), paracetamol, ibuprofen and indomethacin, is mediated predominantly by inhibition of prostaglandin G/H synthetase (cyclo-oxygenase), which reduces autocoid signalling via the synthesis and release of prostaglandins. By decreasing circulating prostaglandins, e.g. prostaglandins E_2 and I_2 (PGE_2, PGI_2) NSAIDs reduce blood flow to inflamed tissue and, thereby, contribute to reduced oedema. This mechanism is also probably associated with the effectiveness of NSAIDs in relieving headache. During inflammation, macrophages release interleukin-1. This pyrogen stimulates increased production of PGE_2 in the hypothalamus which, in turn, raises the set-point body temperature. Again by reducing PGE_2 levels, NSAIDs can be used successfully to lower raised body temperature (antipyretic). Thirdly, NSAIDs can be used to relieve certain types of pain in which prostaglandin signalling is involved. Analgesia is achieved by reducing the prostaglandin-mediated sensitization of nociceptic (pain) nerve endings to inflammatory signals from bradykinin and 5-hydroxytryptamine. NSAIDs may also be used to prevent vascular occlusion as reduced thromboxane A_2 production reduces platelet aggregation.

There are two isoforms of cyclo-oxygenase: cyclo-oxygenase 1 (COX-1) and cyclo-oxygenase 2 (COX-2). COX-1 is expressed constitutively in many tissues, while COX-2 expression is induced by inflammatory stimuli. Current NSAIDs are relatively non-selective for the two COX isoforms and, hence, in addition to their anti-inflammatory actions, several unwanted side-effects occur in the gastrointestinal tract, kidney, central nervous system and haematopoietic system due to the inhibition of COX-1. In each case the side-effects occur as a result of the inhibition of prostaglandin or thromboxane synthesis, important in normal homeostatic control in the tissue. For example, in the gastrointestinal tract, PGE_2 and PGI_2 maintain the integrity of the gastroduodenal mucosa, inhibit acid secretion and modulate blood flow. Inhibition of COX-1 in the gastrointestinal tract by NSAIDs, therefore, leads to gastric irritation, peptic ulcers, bleeding and perforation. These side-effects can be countered by replacement therapy with synthetic prostaglandin. In the kidney, prostaglandins maintain renal blood flow. Again, inhibition of COX-1 by NSAIDs can lead to impaired renal function leading to oedema. Other adverse effects include dizziness, headache, bleeding and skin rashes.

All of the side-effects of NSAIDs are due to inhibition of COX-1 in different tissues and illustrate possible difficulties arising from targeting therapy to an early reaction in a metabolic pathway present in many tissues. Development of a COX-2 selective NSAID may be more desirable to reduce unwanted side-effects.

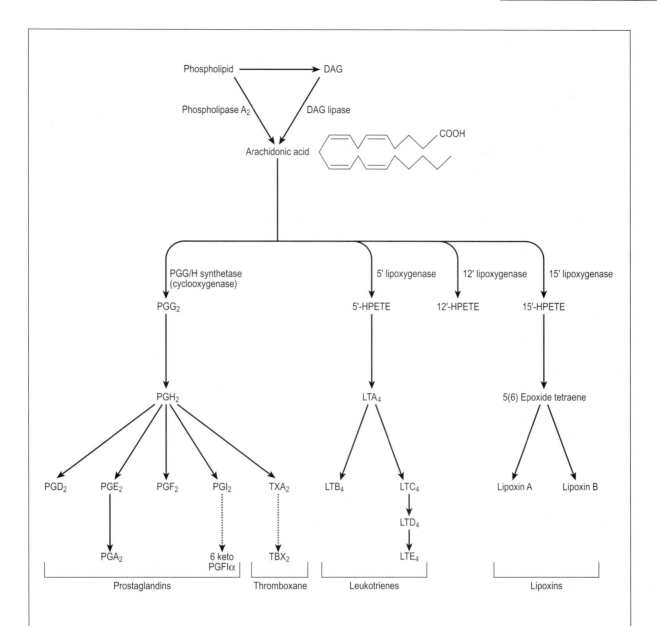

Fig. 7.6 Summary of pathways for the synthesis of eicosanoids from arachidonic acid. Cellular production of eicosanoids is determined by which pathway enzymes are expressed. DAG, 1,2-diacylglycerol; HPETE, hydroperoxyeicosatetraenoic acid; LT, leukotriene; PG, prostaglandin; TX, thromboxane.

Metabolite	Target cells	Response of target tissue
Thromboxane A_2	Platelets	Aggregation
	Vascular smooth muscle	Vasoconstriction
	Bronchial smooth muscle	Bronchoconstriction
Prostaglandin D_2	Platelets	Inhibition of aggregation
	Vascular smooth muscle	Vasodilatation
	Bronchial smooth muscle	Bronchoconstriction
Prostaglandin I_2	Platelets	Inhibition of aggregation
	Vascular smooth muscle	Vasodilatation
Prostaglandin E_2	Vascular smooth muscle	Vasodilatation
	Renal thick ascending limb and collecting tubule	Attenuation of water and NaCl reabsorption in response to vasopressin
Leukotriene B_4	Polymorphonuclear lymphocytes	Chemokinetic, chemotactic, degranulation
	Vascular endothelium	Increased permeability
Leukotrienes C_4, D_4 and E_4	Smooth muscle (intestinal, respiratory and vascular)	Contraction
Lipoxins	Neutrophils, endothelial cells	Inhibit chemotaxis and adhesion

Table 7.1 Arachidonic acid metabolites as extracellular messenger molecules

Ca^{2+} as a second messenger

Cellular Ca^{2+} metabolism

A variety of cellular responses are mediated by changes in the concentration of cytosolic Ca^{2+}, e.g. contraction, secretion, glycogenolysis. By binding to specific binding sites, Ca^{2+} ions induce conformational changes in Ca^{2+}-sensitive proteins, which modulate the activity of the protein. Cells go to great lengths to maintain extremely low (100–200 nM) cytosolic Ca^{2+} concentrations ([Ca^{2+}]$_i$) in spite of the large electrochemical gradient (10 000:1), which favours strongly the influx of Ca^{2+} from the interstitial fluid (1–2 mM). Mechanisms to maintain low [Ca^{2+}]$_i$ probably evolved to prevent insoluble deposits forming with phosphate, which is the main intracellular buffer. Although there is a limited amount of buffering of Ca^{2+} by binding to intracellular proteins, cells need to expend energy to extrude Ca^{2+} through the plasma membrane or to sequester it in intracellular vesicular stores. Indeed, total cell [Ca^{2+}] can be in the millimolar range when stored calcium is taken into account. Extrusion occurs via Ca^{2+}-ATPase and Na$^+$–Ca^{2+} exchangers in the plasma membrane and sequestration into intracellular vesicular stores via a second Ca^{2+}-ATPase (SERCA) (Fig. 7.7). In the lumen of these stores the free [Ca^{2+}] is buffered by binding to low-affinity Ca^{2+}-binding proteins, e.g. calsequestrin. This reduces the unfavourable gradient for further Ca^{2+} uptake and allows a considerable total concentration (in the millimolar range) to be stored. Uptake into mitochondria, driven by the electrochemical proton gradient, can also occur to buffer Ca^{2+} during prolonged periods of significantly raised cytosolic [Ca^{2+}].

Transient 5–10-fold increases in total [Ca^{2+}]$_i$ occur in response to cell activation and may be mediated by influx across the plasma membrane or release from intracellular stores. In both cases the movement of Ca^{2+} across the membrane is driven by the electrochemical gradient through one or more Ca^{2+}-specific ion channels. These may be directly ligand-gated, e.g. plasma membrane N-methyl-D-aspartate (NMDA) receptors and InsP$_3$ receptors in the ER, or may open in response to changes in membrane potential, e.g. voltage-gated Ca^{2+} channels in the plasma membrane (Fig. 7.8). Owing to the limited diffusion of Ca^{2+} in the cytoplasm, Ca^{2+} transients are often localized to microdomains within the cell, e.g. below the plasma membrane, where the [Ca^{2+}]$_i$ may rise to 100–200 μM, e.g. to trigger exocytosis.

Capacitance Ca^{2+} entry

Ca^{2+} mobilized from internal stores may be re-sequestered by the ER or pumped out of the cell by plasma membrane Ca^{2+}-ATPases. In principle this latter mechanism could lead to depletion of the Ca^{2+} store. In practice, reduced lumenal [Ca^{2+}] in the ER (SR) stimulates a refilling of internal Ca^{2+} stores from extracellular sources. Ca^{2+} influx across the plasma membrane is mediated by store-operated Ca^{2+} channels. The Ca^{2+} entering the cell probably enters the cytoplasm before being taken up rapidly by ER structures just beneath the plasma membrane. Such refilling of internal Ca^{2+} stores is known as **capacitance entry** of Ca^{2+}. Whether store depletion is communicated to store-operated Ca^{2+} channels directly by physical coupling or indirectly via a specific chemical messenger is currently an area of active research.

Ca^{2+}-modulated proteins

Ca^{2+}-modulated proteins can be classified into **helix–loop–helix motif** (**HLH** or EF-hand)-containing and non-HLH-containing proteins based on the structure of the Ca^{2+} binding site(s) present. In non-HLH proteins the Ca^{2+} binding site is usually contained in the same polypeptide as the protein activity (e.g. PKC), whereas HLH-containing polypeptides are generally a subunit of an oligomeric protein in which the enzyme or other activity resides in an independent subunit. The major HLH-containing Ca^{2+}-binding protein is **calmodulin**. This small polypeptide contains four HLH motifs in each molecule that are highly selective for Ca^{2+} over Na$^+$, K$^+$ and the most abundant cytoplasmic divalent cation, Mg^{2+}. Large conformational changes in the calmodulin molecule are induced by the successive binding of pairs of Ca^{2+} ions. In most cases interaction of calmodulin with target proteins occurs only after activation of calmodulin by binding Ca^{2+}, although in some cases calmodulin remains tightly bound to the target enzyme even at resting Ca^{2+} concentrations, e.g. glycogen phosphorylase. The Ca^{2+}–calmodulin complex is responsible for the activation of a large number of cellular proteins, e.g. Ca^{2+}–calmodulin-dependent protein kinase (CaM-kinase) and the plasma membrane Ca^{2+}-ATPase. Other HLH-containing proteins are specific for a single oligomeric protein, e.g. tropomyosin C.

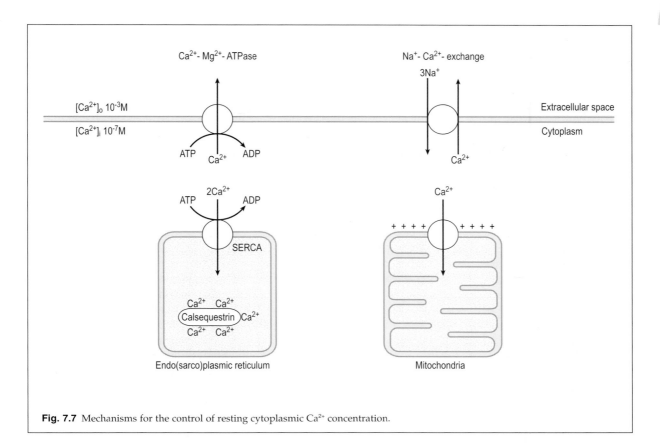

Fig. 7.7 Mechanisms for the control of resting cytoplasmic Ca^{2+} concentration.

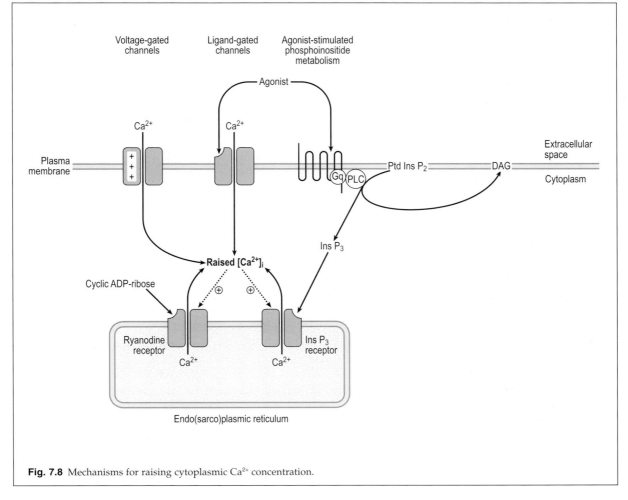

Fig. 7.8 Mechanisms for raising cytoplasmic Ca^{2+} concentration.

Ca²⁺-induced Ca²⁺ release from internal stores, Ca²⁺ oscillations and waves

When observed with Ca²⁺-sensitive dyes, a Ca²⁺ signal may be observed to remain localized to a region of the cytosol near to the plasma membrane, it may spread as a wave of rising $[Ca^{2+}]_i$ across the cell or the cell may even enter a programme of agonist-induced Ca²⁺ oscillations depending on the cell type and the agonist applied. Waves of increased $[Ca^{2+}]_i$ and Ca²⁺ oscillations result from an enhanced release of Ca²⁺ from internal stores in response to an initial local rise in second messenger InsP₃ or $[Ca^{2+}]_i$ (Fig. 7.9). This induced Ca²⁺ release occurs either through opening of the InsP₃ receptor channel in response to second messenger InsP₃ or Ca²⁺ binding on the cytoplasmic face of the receptor or by the activation of a second Ca²⁺-activated Ca²⁺ channel in the ER. This second channel, termed the **ryanodine receptor (RyR)**, is uniquely sensitive to the plant alkaloid ryanodine, which blocks the channel at high concentration. Release of stored Ca²⁺ through ER Ca²⁺ channels in response to a local rise in $[Ca^{2+}]_i$ followed by periods of store refilling result in Ca²⁺ waves or oscillations (Fig. 7.9).

The cardiac cycle

In ventricular muscle, depolarization of the sarcolemma leads to the opening of voltage-gated Ca²⁺ channels and influx of Ca²⁺. This supplies only ~15% of the Ca²⁺ required for contraction. The sarcolemmal Ca²⁺ channels are coupled functionally to Ca²⁺ release channels in the SR such that the local rise in $[Ca^{2+}]_i$ between the sarcolemma and SR triggers release of internal Ca²⁺ stores by Ca²⁺-induced Ca²⁺ release. This supplies the remaining Ca²⁺ required for contraction. During sarcolemmal depolarization, when the driving force on Na⁺ is reduced, Na⁺–Ca²⁺ exchange operates in reverse mode and contributes to the influx of Ca²⁺. As the membrane potential returns to resting levels, Na⁺–Ca²⁺ exchange reverses leading to a reduction in $[Ca^{2+}]_i$ in synergy with the actions of the plasma membrane and SR Ca²⁺-ATPases, which are stimulated by Ca²⁺–calmodulin complex in response to the raised $[Ca^{2+}]_i$.

The use of Ca²⁺ entry blockers in cardiovascular disease

The organic Ca²⁺ entry blockers or Ca²⁺ antagonists are a family of drugs that act selectively on the cardiovascular system. Their action is to block L-type, voltage-gated Ca²⁺ channels and so reduce Ca²⁺ entry into vascular and cardiac cells. This lowers $[Ca^{2+}]_i$ resulting in a reduced contractile activity in vascular and cardiac muscle. The Ca²⁺ antagonists include 1,4-dihydropyridine (e.g. nifedipine), phenylalkylamine (e.g. varapamil) and benzothiazepine (e.g. diltiazem) drug groups. At therapeutic concentrations, nifedipine exerts its major effect in vascular smooth muscle without much effect in the heart. Verapamil and diltiazem, in addition, also affect Ca²⁺ channels in cardiac tissue. This tissue selectivity is useful in targeting therapeutic effect.

The Ca²⁺ antagonists find wide application in the treatment of vascular disorders. Use of dihydropyridines is indicated in **hypertension** to lower vascular smooth muscle tone and hence blood pressure because of their vascular selectivity. Ca²⁺ antagonists are also effective in **Raynaud's disease** in which intense vasoconstriction occurs in the arteries supplying fingers and toes in response to cold and vibration. To treat the **ischaemic heart** in **angina**, dihydropyridines and diltiazem can be given to improve the coronary circulation, by reducing coronary artery contraction, and to reduce cardiac oxygen consumption, by reducing contratile activity. At higher doses, the Ca²⁺ antagonists can block atrioventricular impulse conduction. Verapamil may be used, therefore, in the treatment of **supraventricular dysrhythmias**.

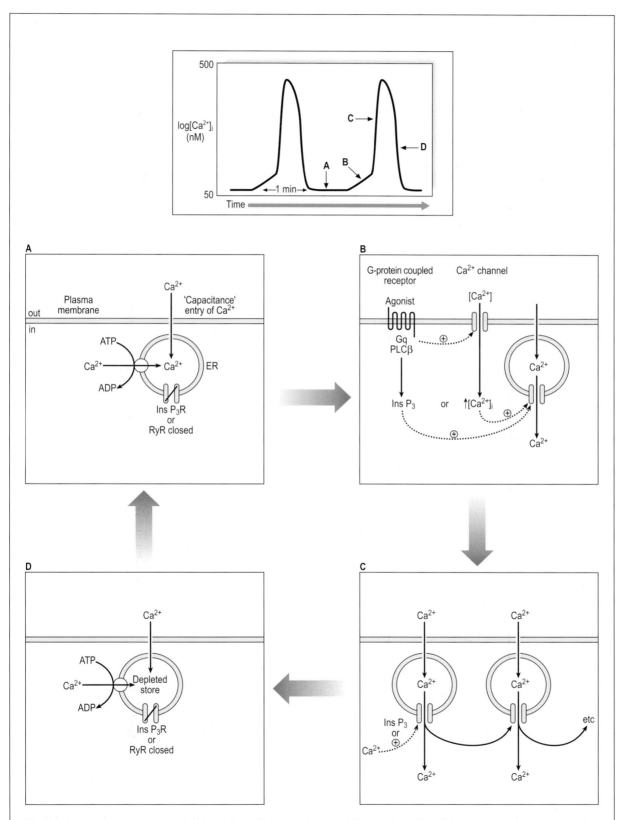

Fig. 7.9 Proposed mechanisms underlying Ca^{2+} oscillations and waves. (**A**) In resting cells Ca^{2+} is taken up by internal stores by sarco(endo)plasmic reticulum Ca^{2+}-ATPase (SERCA) and 'capacitance' entry down the concentration gradient. (**B**) Stimulation of the cell resulting in an increase in $InsP_3$ or $[Ca^{2+}]_i$ results in Ca^{2+} release from internal stores via $InsP_3$-receptor ($InsP_3R$) or ryanodine-receptor (RyR) channels. (**C**) The rise in $[Ca^{2+}]_i$ triggers further Ca^{2+}-induced Ca^{2+} release from adjacent stores until (**D**) store depletion results in channel closing and refilling of internal stores. When the stores are replete, the raised lumenal $[Ca^{2+}]$ sensitizes the Ca^{2+} release channels such that they may open spontaneously or may respond to second messengers ($InsP_3$, $InsP_3R$; cyclic ADP-ribose, RyR; Ca^{2+}, $InsP_3R$ and RyR) to produce a second Ca^{2+} spike. ER, endoplasmic reticulum; $PLC\beta$, phospholipase $C\beta$.

Kinases and phosphatases in cell signalling

Regulation of enzyme and protein activity is often achieved by phosphorylation or dephosphorylation, the directed covalent modification of the protein by the transfer onto or removal of a phosphate moiety, respectively. The introduction or removal of a negatively charged phosphate group at specific residues in the target protein brings about an alteration in the conformation of the polypeptide that can cause either an activation or inhibition depending on the protein. Protein phosphorylation is catalysed by a family of protein kinases that transfer the terminal phosphate from ATP onto the target residue. Dephosphorylation is catalysed by a family of protein phosphatases that facilitate the hydrolysis of the phosphate bond.

Protein kinases

Protein kinases may be classified, according to the amino acid residue they phosphorylate, into **serine (threonine) kinases** and **tyrosine kinases**. Most target proteins are phosphorylated on serine or threonine residues. Tyrosine phosphorylation may only constitute about 0.1% of all protein phosphorylation events. Further specificity is governed predominantly by the nature of the amino acid residues around the phosphorylation site, although secondary and tertiary structure are known to be important.

Regulation of kinase activity

All protein kinases have regulatory and catalytic elements. These may be contained on separate polypeptide subunits (e.g. cA-PK) (Fig. 7.10) or combined in a single polypeptide (e.g. PKC) (Fig. 7.11). In the absence of regulator molecules, protein kinases are inactive. They may be activated by interaction between the regulator molecule and the regulatory element or by undergoing a conformational change to render the catalytic site accessible to substrate.

Activation of protein kinases by second messengers

Several second messengers interact with specific protein kinases in order to elicit, at least part of, their action in the cell (e.g. cyclic AMP, cyclic GMP, DAG, Ca^{2+}). For example, cyclic AMP binds to the two regulatory subunits of tetrameric protein kinase A (cA-PK, PKA) to release two catalytic subunits (Fig. 7.10). The released catalytic subunits are, thereby, activated and go on to phosphorylate a specific subset of proteins in the cell defined by the recognition of a defining structure of susceptible phosphorylation sites. Where a subset of cellular proteins is modulated by a single kinase, the result is for protein activities to be modulated in concert. For example, in hepatic glycogen metabolism, breakdown is increased while synthesis is reduced in response to cA-PK activation producing a concerted mobilization of glucose (see Fig. 7.2).

Multiple phosphorylation of target proteins

Many target proteins present more than one phosphorylation site. These may represent multiple sites for a single protein kinase, specific sites for different kinases or may be sites phosphorylated by more than one kinase. Phosphorylation of at least one site will result in an alteration of protein activity. Phosphorylation at multiple sites may alter the activity of the protein but could also modulate the response to phosphorylation at one of the other sites or modify the ability of the target to be phosphorylated at another site. Clearly, the potential for integration of responses to several signalling pathways is possible, depending on the target protein in question.

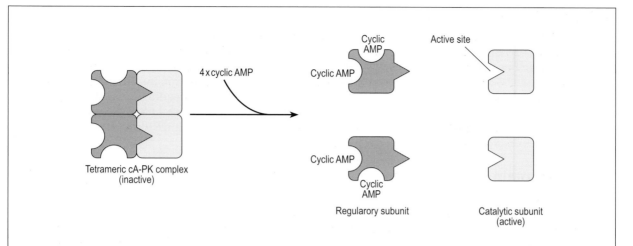

Fig. 7.10 Activation of cyclic AMP-dependent protein kinase (cA-PK) by cyclic AMP. Binding of cyclic AMP to the regulatory subunits decreases their affinity for the catalytic subunits and releases them from pseudosubstrate inhibition in the inactive tetrameric complex.

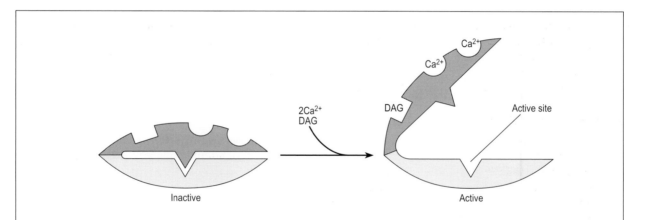

Fig. 7.11 Activation of protein kinase C (PKC). A conformational change in PKC in response to binding of diacylglycerol (DAG) releases the pseudosubstrate from the active site and removes the inhibition of activity. Ca^{2+} binding acts in synergy to activate the enzyme. Note: there are multiple isoforms of PKC some of which are not activated as above. The PKC family can be subdivided into Ca^{2+}-sensitive, 'classic' (α,β,γ), Ca^{2+}-insensitive, 'novel' ($\delta,\epsilon,\eta,\theta$), and 'atypical' ($\lambda,\zeta$) forms. No regulators have been characterized for the atypical PKCs.

Autophosphorylation of kinases

Most protein kinases are also able to phosphorylate themselves on serine, threonine or tyrosine residues. This intramolecular reaction is termed **autophosphorylation** and is important for self-regulation. For example, autophosphorylation of Ca^{2+}–calmodulin-dependent protein kinase abolishes the calmodulin-dependence of the enzyme and autophosphorylation of the insulin receptor kinase results in an activation of the kinase, which is then independent of the binding of insulin. Autophosphorylation plays a further important role in the tyrosine kinase-linked receptors as phosphotyrosine residues resulting from receptor autophosphorylation provide interaction sites for effector molecules and transducing proteins (see Figs 6.6 and 6.10).

Phosphoprotein phosphatases

Like the kinases, protein phosphatases can be classified on the basis of their specificity for the hydrolysis of phosphorylated residues into serine (threonine) and tyrosine phosphatases. Several types of **serine (threonine)-phosphoprotein phosphatases** (Table 7.2) and a large number of different **tyrosine-phosphoprotein phosphatases** have been characterized. The latter are found both as cytoplasmic and as membrane-bound enzymes. The membrane-bound tyrosine phosphatases are probably receptors activated by interaction of an agonist or ligand and have been implicated in intracellular signalling in response to adhesion proteins and antigen in leucocytes.

Cross-talk between signalling pathways

The signalling pathways described above do not operate independently of each other, rather there is considerable **cross-talk** between them. Cross-talk mechanisms allow the level of activity in a pathway to be modulated by the activity in parallel pathways. This permits a cell to integrate its response to multiple extracellular signals and, thus, to produce an appropriate overall response. The exact nature of the response in any cell will depend partly on the size of each external signal but also on the nature of the signalling pathway components present in the cell. For example, eight isoforms of adenylyl cyclase have been characterized. Differential sensitivity and responses to Ca^{2+}, G-protein $\beta\gamma$ subunit complexes and kinases are possible depending on the isoform of adenylyl cyclase that is expressed by the cell (Table 7.3).

Targeting proteins for components of signalling pathways: molecular scaffolds

It is becoming clear that, rather than being totally free within the cytoplasm, several kinases and phosphatases may be compartmentalized within the cell by subcellular targeting proteins associated with membrane structures. Targeted localization of kinases and phosphatases can have the effect of increasing the selectivity of broad-specificity kinases or phosphatases by favouring their access to particular substrates. Several anchoring proteins have been characterized that localize kinases and phosphatases to different cellular localizations. Further complexity is possible when the targeting protein is able to bind several kinases and/or phosphatases providing a **molecular scaffold** to localize signalling enzymes. An example of a **scaffold protein** is A-kinase anchoring protein 79 (AKAP79), which targets cA-PK, PKC and protein phosphatase-2B to the postsynaptic density of mammalian synapses. In this way molecular scaffolds can provide for the integrated response of an effector to several second messenger pathways.

Property	PP-1	PP-2A	PP-2B*	PP-2C
Preference for phosphorylase kinase α or β subunit	β	α	α	α
Dependence on divalent cations	No	No	Ca^{2+}	Mg^{2+}
Dependence on calmodulin	No	No	Yes	No
Inhibited by inhibitor-1 and -2	Yes	No	No	No
Inhibited by okadaic acid	+++	+++++	+	−
Cellular localization	Associated with intracellular structures[a]	Broad distribution	Broad distribution	Broad distribution

Table 7.2 Protein (serine/threonine) phosphatases (PP). [a]Examples of intracellular PP-1 associations: Glycogen, PP-1G, SR, PP-1SR; Myofibrils, PP-1M; soluble, PP-1l

Subtype	Effect of Ca^{2+}	Stimulation by $G_s\alpha$	Inhibition by $G_i\alpha$	Effect of βγ complex	Stimulation by PKC
I	Stimulation	Mild	Yes	Inhibition	No
III	Stimulation	Yes	?	None	No
VIII	Stimulation	Mild	?	?	No
II	No	Yes	No	Stimulation	Yes
IV	No	Yes	?	Stimulation	No
VII	No	Yes	?	?	Yes
V	Inhibition	Yes	Yes	None	No
VI	Inhibition	Yes	Yes	None	No

Table 7.3 Properties of isoforms of adenylyl cyclase (adapted from Cooper et al. 1995 Nature 374: 421–424)

Desensitization (tachyphylaxis) in signalling pathways

When cells are exposed continuously to an extracellular messenger or drug they can often become increasingly resistant to stimulation (Fig. 7.12). This loss of sensitivity is known as **desensitization** or **tachyphylaxis** when it occurs acutely over a few minutes and **tolerance** or **resistance** when occurring over a period of days or weeks. Desensitisation takes two forms (Fig. 7.13):

- When sensitivity is lost to a single extracellular agonist, this is known as **homologous desensitization**
- When sensitivity is lost to multiple stimulating agonists in response to the presence of a single stimulating agonist, this is known as **heterologous desensitization**.

Many mechanisms may contribute to cellular desensitization. At the level of the receptor, a change in receptor properties or a reduction in the number of receptors may bring about desensitization. Alternatively, a metabolic desensitization could occur through an exhaustion of mediator within the signalling pathway, an increased degradation of the extracellular signalling molecule and/or physiological adaptation to the raised levels of signalling molecule.

Receptor desensitization

Ligand-gated ion channels desensitize rapidly. Within the time scale of channel opening and closing, when continually exposed to agonist, the receptors undergo a slow transition to a stable conformation that binds agonist with high affinity but in which the channel remains closed. Desensitization is reversed when the concentration of agonist falls and the receptor changes conformation to a lower-affinity state allowing the bound agonist to dissociate.

Desensitization of **G-protein-linked receptors** can occur through modification of the receptor by phosphorylation, a reversible removal of the receptor from the plasma membrane or an irreversible removal and degradation of the receptor, known as **down-regulation** (Fig. 7.14). Receptor phosphorylation may be in response to second messenger activated kinases (e.g. cA-PK, PKC) or specific G-protein receptor protein kinases (GRKs), e.g. β-adrencoceptor protein kinase (βARK).

Desensitization of activated receptors by receptor-mediated endocytosis occurs over a slower time scale (Fig. 7.14C). If the internalized receptors are sorted and recycled to the plasma membrane, this results in a short desensitization. However, on prolonged cell stimulation, receptors may become lysosomally targeted where they are degraded, resulting in receptor down-regulation. The results of down-regulation are reversed only by the synthesis of new receptors. It is noteworthy that down-regulation of receptors can occur in response to molecules other than agonist. For example, ethanol and barbiturates, which are not receptor agonists, may lead to down-regulation of G-protein-coupled receptors, an example of **tolerance**.

Receptor desensitization and insulin resistance in diabetes

In non-insulin dependent (type II) diabetes, tissues become resistant to insulin even though insulin may be present at raised levels. One contributory factor to insulin resistance is the down-regulation of insulin receptors.

Drug habituation

Down-regulation in general may explain habituation to drug therapy.

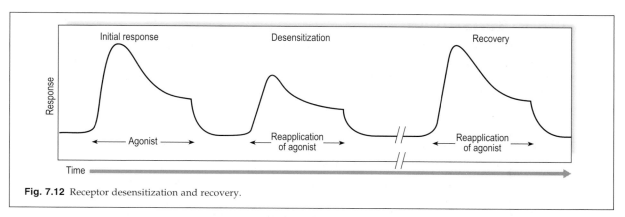

Fig. 7.12 Receptor desensitization and recovery.

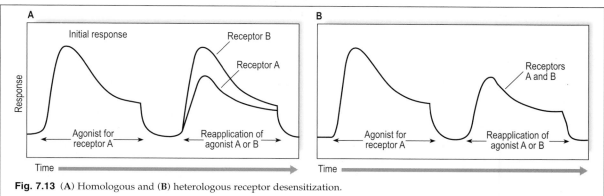

Fig. 7.13 (**A**) Homologous and (**B**) heterologous receptor desensitization.

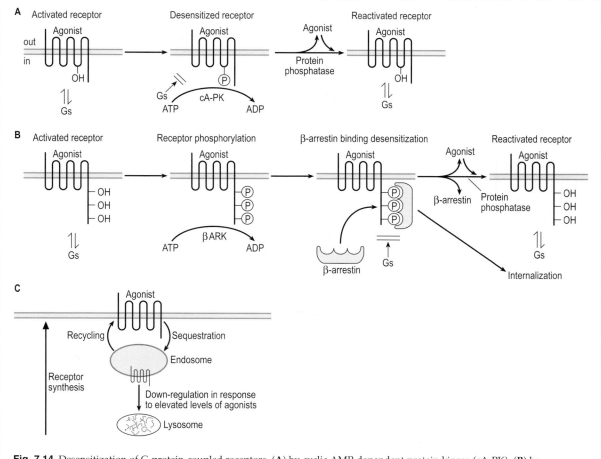

Fig. 7.14 Desensitization of G-protein-coupled receptors, (**A**) by cyclic AMP-dependent protein kinase (cA-PK), (**B**) by β-adrenoceptor protein kinase (β-ARK) and (**C**) by receptor-mediated endocytosis.

Cell supersensitivity

The sensitivity of a cell to an external stimulus may be increased by convergent cross-talk between signalling pathways. For example, glucagon and glucagon-like peptide do not stimulate release of insulin from β-cells per se but potentiate the response to a given level of glucose through a cA-PK mechanism. Similarly, β-adrenergic stimulation in the heart can increase heart rate and force of contraction again through a cA-PK mechanism via phosphorylation of L-type voltage-sensitive Ca^{2+} channels. This phosphorylation increases the probability that Ca^{2+} channels will open and, therefore, leads to a greater Ca^{2+} signal for a given depolarization.

Supersensitivity may also occur following interruption of normal signalling to the cell. This is often seen after denervation of peripheral tissues. The response in the postsynaptic cell can be to increase the number of receptors and to increase postjunctional responsiveness by increasing electrical excitability, even in the absence of additional receptors. Loss of mechanisms for the removal of transmitter from synapses, e.g. reduced noradrenaline uptake in adrenergic synapses and reduced cholinesterase in cholinergic synapses, can make a substantial contribution to postsynaptic cell supersensitivity after denervation.

'Rebound' effects on removal of drug therapy

Supersensitivity is an important consideration when removing therapy that has been given for some time. Adaptive responses in cells in an attempt to overcome the drug effect during treatment may result in a 'rebound' effect in response to natural agonists when therapy ceases. For example, sudden withdrawal of β-adrenoceptor antagonists can cause an increased sympathetic stimulation of the heart. The resulting increase in heart rate and force of contraction, and hence oxygen consumption, can lead to the development of angina pectoris and myocardial infarction. Where β-adrenoceptor antagonist therapy is to be withdrawn, it is recommended that this is done gradually.

Further reading

Barritt G J 1992 Communication within animal cells. Oxford University Press, Oxford

Bootman M D, Berridge M J 1995 The elemental principles of calcium signaling. Cell 83: 675–678

Clapham D E 1995 Calcium signaling. Cell 80: 259–268

Faux M C, Scott J D 1996 More on target with protein-phosphorylation – conferring specificity by location. Trends in Biochemical Sciences 21: 312–315

Hardie D G 1991 Biochemical messengers: hormones, neurotransmitters and growth factors. Chapman and Hall, London

Pawson T 1995 Protein modules and signalling networks. Nature 373: 572–580

Revision questions

1. What are the criteria by which the cyclic nucleotides can be considered as 'second messengers'?

2. How can receptor stimulation of phosphatidylinositol polyphosphate hydrolysis give rise to more than one second messenger?

3. How is resting intracellular Ca^{2+} ion concentration ($[Ca^{2+}]_i$) maintained? What mechanisms exist for raising $[Ca^{2+}]_i$?

4. What is the function of calmodulin in transducing a Ca^{2+} signal to other cellular components?

5. Many second messengers ultimately control the activity of a protein kinase. Because cellular activation results from protein phosphorylation in each case, how is specificity of hormone, local mediator or neurotransmitter action preserved?

6. What is the difference between homologous and heterologous desensitization?

7. Describe mechanisms by which adrenoceptors may become desensitized?

8. How may cells develop supersensitivity to extracellular signalling molecules?

Answers to revision questions

1. The cyclic nucleotides, cyclic AMP and cyclic GMP, are maintained at low cellular concentrations and are only produced in response to appropriate receptor stimulation. The level of cyclic nucleotides produced and the tissue response are proportional to the extracellular signal. Finally, cyclic nucleotides are degraded rapidly.

2. Phospholipase cleavage of $PtdInsP_2$ releases the second messengers $InsP_3$ and DAG, which act on $InsP_3$ receptors to release stored Ca^{2+} and PKC, respectively. Ca^{2+} is also a second messenger and acts on Ca^{2+}-sensitive proteins. $InsP_3$-kinase may also phosphorylate $InsP_3$ to produce $InsP_4$, itself implicated as a second messenger enhancing Ca^{2+} uptake.

3. Resting $[Ca^{2+}]_i$ is maintained by Ca^{2+} buffering by intracellular proteins, extrusion through PMCA and Na^+–Ca^{2+} exchange and sequestration into vesicular stores by SERCA. $[Ca^{2+}]_i$ may be raised by Ca^{2+} entry through ligand- or voltage-gated Ca^{2+} channels or release of stored Ca^{2+} in response to $InsP_3$ and/or Ca^{2+}.

4. Calmodulin is a specific Ca^{2+}-binding protein with high selectivity over Na^+, K^+ and Mg^{2+}. Binding of Ca^{2+} induces a large conformational change, which permits activation of target proteins by the Ca^{2+}-calmodulin complex.

5. Specific protein kinases are activated in response to different intracellular signalling pathways. Each kinase has a restricted substrate specificity defined by the amino acid sequence around phosphorylated residues. Thus, signal specificity is maintained through to the cellular processes activated or inhibited by kinase activation.

6. Homologous desensitization occurs when sensitivity is lost to a single agonist. Heterologous desensitization occurs when sensitivity is lost to several different stimulating agonists in response to the presence of a single agonist.

7. Adrenoceptors may become desensitized as a result of phosphorylation of the receptor on the cytoplasmic side of the membrane. Where phosphorylation is mediated by β-adrenoceptor kinase, the subsequent binding of β-arrestin stimulates removal of the receptor from the membrane by endocytosis. Degradation of receptor in response to high levels of agonist results in a more prolonged down-regulation of receptor number.

8. Supersensitivity in signalling pathways may arise as a result of potentiating cross-talk from other signalling pathways. It may also be caused by adaptive responses to interrupted cell signalling pathways, for example when drug therapy is terminated, producing 'rebound effects'.

Signal transduction: electrical signalling

Using a very fine micropipette (microelectrode) to penetrate the plasma membrane of a cell allows the electrical potential across the plasma membrane to be measured. All cells have an electrical potential difference across their plasma membrane (**membrane potential**) and this is expressed as the voltage inside relative to that on the outside of the membrane. Animal cells have resting membrane potentials ranging from approximately −20 to −90 mV depending on the cell type and changes in this potential difference form the basis of electrical signalling in cells.

The resting membrane potential

At rest, cell membranes are more permeable to K^+ ions than other ionic species because of facilitated diffusion through K^+ channel proteins which form K^+-specific pores in the membrane. The extracellular and intracellular K^+ concentrations in a 'typical' cell are 4.5 mM and 160 mM, respectively; therefore, K^+ tends to move outwards down its concentration gradient. Since large protein anions inside the cell are unable to follow K^+ out of the cell, a negative potential develops on the intracellular face of the plasma membrane. This growing potential difference then opposes the further efflux of K^+ ions. An equilibrium is reached when the diffusional and electrical forces are balanced and there is no net movement of K^+ ions. At equilibrium, the potential across the membrane is termed the **potassium equilibrium potential** (E_K) (Fig. 8.1). Equilibrium potentials can be calculated (Table 8.1).

Although the passage of K^+ ions through K^+ channels predominates in the resting cell, the resting membrane potential never reaches E_K. This is because the plasma membrane is not totally impermeable to other ions and the passage of these ions through selective ion channels contributes to the overall membrane potential (Fig. 8.2). Note: Only very few ions need to move across the plasma membrane to establish a membrane potential.

Increased membrane excitability in hyperkalaemia

The consequences of **hyperkalaemia**, where the extracellular concentration of K^+ is raised, are a more positive E_K and, hence, a more positive resting membrane potential. Cellular electrical activity depends on the ability to depolarize membranes (see below). Thus, in the heart in hyperkalaemia, a lesser change in ion conductance is required to depolarize and so excite cardiac membranes. The result of this increased excitability is ventricular arrhythmia, which can lead to fibrillation and, if left untreated, can be life-threatening.

Changing the membrane potential

Changing the permeability of the plasma membrane to a particular ion can cause a change in the membrane potential. Opening an ion channel for any ion results in the movement of the membrane potential towards the equilibrium potential for that ion (see Table 8.1). Thus, opening K^+ or Cl^- channels results in an increase in membrane potential with the inside of the cell becoming more negative (Fig. 8.3). This is termed **hyperpolarization**. Conversely, opening Na^+ or Ca^{2+} channels results in a decrease in membrane potential with the inside becoming less negative. This is termed **depolarization**. Channels can exist in three major states: open, closed or inactivated (see Fig. 8.4C). Alterations in the opening or closing of different ion channels via their **gating mechanisms** allow the membrane potential of the cell to be changed. Channel gating occurs by two main mechanisms:

- **ligand-gating**, where binding of a ligand to a receptor site on the channel results in channel opening (or closing). The ligand may be an extracellular signalling molecule or an intracellular messenger, depending on the channel type (see Chapter 6)
- **voltage-gating**, where the channel opens or closes in response to changes in the membrane potential.

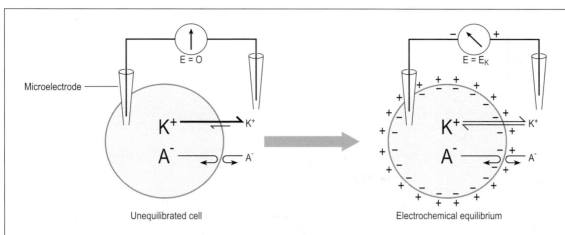

Fig. 8.1 Development of the resting membrane potential. In this example K⁺ is the sole membrane permeant ion and the resting membrane potential (E_K) is attained when the cells come to electrochemical equilibrium with the medium.

Ion	External Concentration (mM)	Internal Concentration (mM)	Equilibrium potential (37°C) (mM)
K⁺	4.5	160	−95
Na⁺	145	10	+71
Ca²⁺	1	0.0001	+122
Cl⁻	114	3	−96

Table 8.1 Calculation of equilibrium potentials. Given the extracellular and intracellular concentrations, the equilibrium potentials for the major membrane permeant ion in a 'typical' cell can be calculated from the **Nernst Equation**:

$$E_{ion} = \frac{RT}{zF} \ln \frac{[ion]_{out}}{[ion]_{in}}$$

where R = the gas constant, T = the absolute temperature, F = Faraday's number and z = valency (+1 for K⁺, −1 for Cl⁻ etc.); $[ion]_{out}$ and $[ion]_{in}$ are the extracellular and intracellular concentrations of the ion

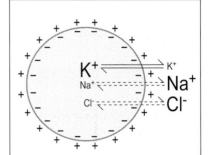

Fig. 8.2 The resting membrane potential is determined by the contribution of the relative permeabilities of several permeant ions.

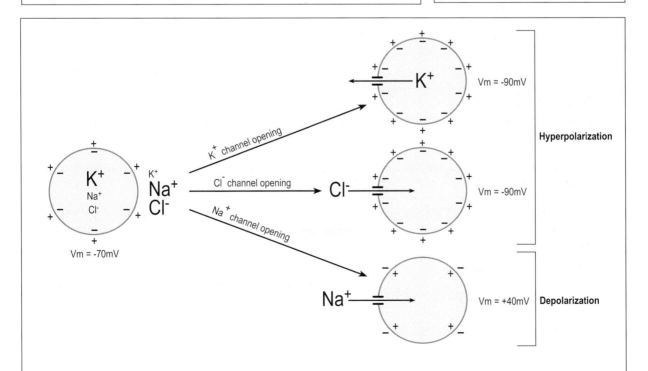

Fig. 8.3 Increasing membrane permeability to a single ionic species can modify the membrane potential V_m.

The action potential

The action potential is the means by which electrical signals are propagated over the plasma membrane of electrically excitable cells. During the action potential the membrane depolarizes briefly before repolarizing to the resting condition (Fig. 8.4). The depolarizing phase of the action potential is generated by an increase in membrane permeability to Na^+ ions through the opening of voltage-gated Na^+ channels. The flow of Na^+ inwards, down its electrochemical gradient, drives the membrane potential towards the equilibrium potential for Na^+ (E_{Na}), thereby depolarizing the membrane. During the repolarization phase of the action potential, Na^+ channels close again, or **inactivate**, reducing the rate of Na^+ influx back to resting levels.

In addition to the inactivation of Na^+ channels in most cells, voltage-gated K^+ channels with slower activation kinetics than Na^+ channels (delayed rectifier channels, K_{DR}) open. The resulting efflux of K^+ down its electrochemical gradient contributes to the repolarization of the membrane and, in some cells, e.g. in nerve axons, the membrane potential can hyperpolarize to a value more negative than the original resting potential before returning once again to the resting membrane potential at which the K^+ channels close.

The duration of an action potential in nerve axon and skeletal muscle is approximately 0.5–1 ms. Longer-duration action potentials (approximately 100 ms) are seen in cardiac ventricular muscle owing to the opening of Ca^{2+} channels with relatively slow activation and inactivation kinetics and closure of inward rectifier K^+ channels.

Initiation of an action potential

Initiation of an action potential depends on the membrane potential rising above a threshold value (approximately –50 mV) at which the inward current just balances the resting outward K^+ conductance. This may occur through (i) an increased open probability (P_O) of voltage-gated Na^+ or Ca^{2+} channels, which leads to membrane depolarization, to exceed the resting K^+ efflux which is hyperpolarizing or (ii) the closure of K^+ channels, which reduces the hyperpolarizing influence on the membrane allowing the membrane potential to rise. As a consequence of the threshold for initiation, action potentials are all-or-nothing. The progress of a wave of depolarization over a cell membrane is then caused by the self-reinforcing way in which Na^+ channels open, i.e. the depolarizing phase of an action potential at one point on the cell membrane will raise the membrane potential in adjacent regions of the membrane sufficiently to exceed the threshold for action potential initiation in that region (Fig. 8.5).

Inactivation of voltage-gated cation channels

Voltage-gated channels pass from closed, through open, to inactivated states on depolarization. Once in the inactivated state a channel cannot reopen until it has been 're-primed' by movement of the membrane potential back to negative values. Thus, once inactivated, Na^+ channels cannot be re-opened during an action potential. This property is important because it prevents irreversible depolarization of the membrane, permits directionality to nerve impulse conduction (Fig. 8.5) and also allows information to be coded with respect to the frequency at which action potentials are fired. Directly after the onset of an action potential there is an **absolute refractory period**, during which the membrane cannot be further excited, followed by a **relative refractory period**, during which it becomes progressively easier to elicit a further action potential as the Na^+ channels recover from inactivation (Fig. 8.6).

Action of local anaesthetics

Local anaesthetics, such as procaine, act on Na^+ channels both as blockers and on gating mechanisms to hold the channel in an inactivated state.

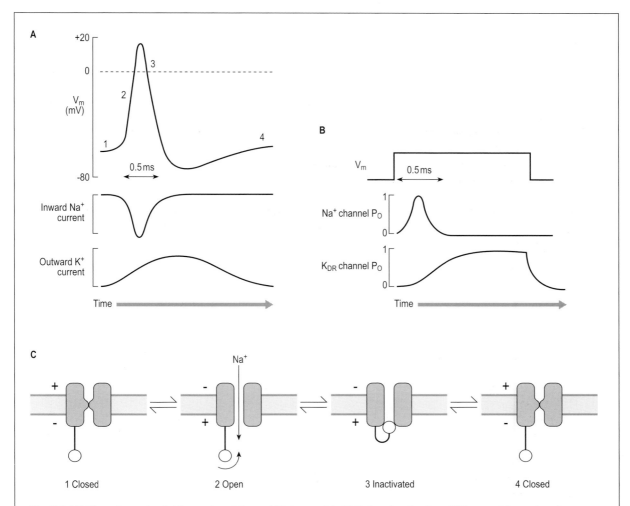

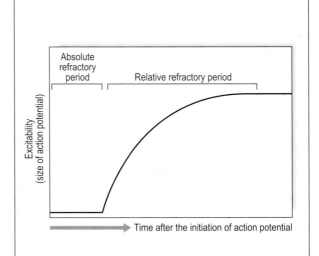

Fig. 8.4 (**A**) The action potential (upper trace). Inward Na$^+$ current (middle trace) and outward K$^+$ current (lower trace) contribute to changes in membrane potential (V$_m$ upper trace) during the action potential in electrically unclamped cells. (**B**) Open probability (P$_O$) of Na$^+$ channels (middle trace) and delayed rectifier K$^+$ (K$_{DR}$) channels (lower trace) underlying the action potential response to a square wave depolarization (upper trace) imposed under voltage-clamp conditions (see Appendix 4). (**C**) Conformational state of voltage-gated Na$^+$ channels at different stages of the action potential (panel a, upper trace). Note: the amount of Na$^+$ and K$^+$ ions that move during the action potential is very small. In the smallest nerve fibres the intracellular Na$^+$ concentration rises by less than 1% and by much less in larger cells.

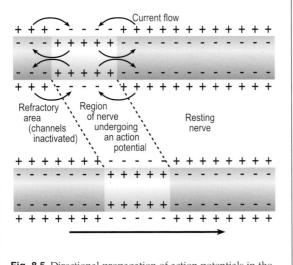

Fig. 8.5 Directional propagation of action potentials in the nerve. Local currents raise the adjacent resting region to threshold, resulting in firing of an action potential.

Fig. 8.6 Excitability of nerve membrane following an action potential.

Ion channels

Structure/function relationships in voltage-gated cation channels

Voltage-gated (also known as voltage-operated or voltage-sensitive) cation channels share a common basic design (Fig. 8.7). The current model proposes a core structure of six hydrophobic membrane-spanning segments (S1–S6) with the N- and C-terminals located on the cytoplasmic side of the membrane (Fig. 8.7A). The major **pore-forming** region (H5, SS1–SS2) is formed by the linking sequence between segments S5 and S6, which is thought to be folded back into the membrane as a hairpin loop of β-sheet. Four of these structures are required to constitute a channel pore (Fig. 8.7B).

Ion selectivity is determined largely by residues in the H5 loop (Fig. 8.7A). This has been demonstrated by site-directed mutagenesis on K^+ channels and the conversion of a Na^+ channel into a Ca^{2+} channel by changing just a single residue in one of the four repeats.

Voltage-sensitivity is conferred by the S4 transmembrane segment (**voltage sensor**), which contains a positively charged residue (lysine or arginine) at every third position in the primary sequence (Fig. 8.7A). The outward movement of this segment in response to the electrical force imposed by membrane depolarization is thought to drive the opening of voltage-gated channels.

Inactivation. In those voltage-gated K^+ channels that inactivate rapidly, an **inactivation 'ball'** located at the N-terminal of the primary structure is thought to swing up on a 'chain' of N-terminal domain amino acid sequence into a vestibule 'ball acceptor' domain in the cytoplasmic mouth of the pore (S4–S5) (Fig. 8.7A). This form of inactivation is termed **N-type inactivation**. Cytoplasmic loop structures constitute the 'ball' in voltage-sensitive Na^+ and Ca^{2+} channels (Fig. 8.7C). It should be noted that a second relatively rapid form of inactivation, **C-type**, has been characterized in some K^+ channels.

Na^+ channel mutations in myotonia

Several forms of **myotonia** (increased muscle excitability and contractility) have been associated with point mutations in the Na^+ channel. These include hyperkalaemic periodic paralysis (HYPP), paramyotonia congenita (PC) and potassium-aggravated myotonia (PAM), for each of which several specific mutations have been identified.

K^+ channel mutations in long QT syndrome

Long QT syndrome is an inherited cardiac arrhythmia in which repolarization of the ventricle is delayed, resulting in a prolonged QT interval in the electrocardiogram. Genetic analysis has revealed mutations in a cardiac muscle delayed rectifier K^+ channel in this condition.

Voltage-insensitive cation channels

Voltage-insensitive K^+ channels contain a pore-forming structure similar to that in voltage-sensitive K^+ channels (Fig. 8.7D) but lack a voltage sensor. These channels are important in maintenance of the resting membrane potential.

Renal epithelial Na^+ channels and hypertension

Liddle's disease is a rare form of hypertension resulting from mutated renal epithelial Na^+ channels. These channels are composed of three subunits ($\alpha\beta\gamma$), each containing two transmembrane segments with cytoplasmic N- and C-terminal domains. Mutations in the C-terminal domains of the β or γ subunits result in a constitutive activation of the Na^+ channel. The resulting excessive Na^+ reabsorbtion from kidney tubules increases water retention and causes an increased blood pressure. Similarly, hypertension resulting from raised aldosterone levels in the rare syndromes of **glucocorticoid-remediable aldosteronism** and **apparent mineralocorticoid excess** is a consequence of increased activity of renal epithelial Na^+ channels.

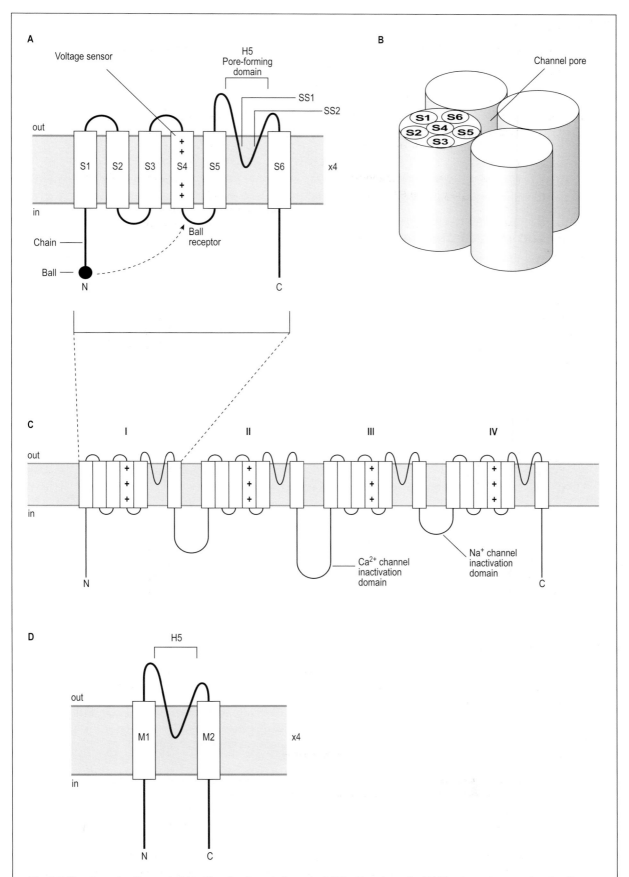

Fig. 8.7 Structure of voltage-gated (**A–C**) and voltage-independent (**D**) cation channels. (**A**) Membrane topography of voltage-gated K^+ channels. (**B**) Arrangement of pore-forming subunits to form a channel. (**C**) Membrane topography of Na^+ and Ca^{2+} channels. (**D**) Membrane topography of voltage-independent, inward rectifier K^+ channels.

Chloride channels

A family of anion-selective channels (CLC) that conduct Cl⁻ ions predominantly, have important functions in cell volume regulation, NaCl movement in kidney tubules and a background hyperpolarizing Cl⁻ current in skeletal muscle.

> **Cl⁻ channel mutations in myotonia**
>
> Point mutations in the skeletal muscle CLC-1 isoform that reduce Cl⁻ conductance and, thereby, increase muscle excitability have been characterized in patients with inherited myotonias (muscle stiffness) such as myotonia congenita or Thomsen's disease and generalized myotonia or Becker's disease.

Auxiliary subunits of channels

In addition to the wide variety of pore-forming polypeptides that make up channels, it is becoming clear that several channels are hetero-oligomers, in which accessory subunits play important roles in determining the kinetic properties of the channel. For example, β subunits in voltage-gated K⁺ channels can be important in determining inactivation kinetics (Fig. 8.8). Accessory subunits can also be important for targeting the pore-forming components to their membrane location. Interactions with the cytoskeleton may also be made to ensure channels localize to appropriate sites, e.g. Na⁺ channels in the nodes of Ranvier (see below).

ATP-binding cassette proteins

Members of the **ATP-binding cassette (ABC) transporter protein** family are important in the modulation of some channels, including the cystic fibrosis transmembrane conductance regulator (or CFTR channel) and the sulphonylurea receptor (see below).

> **Cystic fibrosis transmembrane conductance regulator**
>
> The CFTR Cl⁻ conducting channel was identified as the gene product responsible for cystic fibrosis. It opens in response to phosphorylation in the regulatory region by cA-PK. Cl⁻ efflux from epithelial cells of the lung and secretory ducts of the pancreas is followed by water movement. In cystic fibrosis, several point mutations in the CFTR gene result in defective Cl⁻ transport. The resulting reduction in outward water movement is responsible for the production of an abnormally thick mucous secretion in the small airways of the lung and impaired pancreatic function. In the lung, this can lead to difficulty in breathing and at both sites this abnormality leads to inflammatory responses, infection and progressive damage, which are likely to be fatal.

> **P-glycoprotein and multidrug resistance**
>
> Another notable member of the ABC protein family is the P-glycoprotein, multidrug resistance 1 (MDR1) protein, which acts to extrude drugs from cells. The activity of this protein in cancerous cells is a major cause of resistance to chemical anticancer agents.

Channel modulation

Channel activity may be modulated in response to activation of parallel signalling pathways (Table 8.2). Often this occurs by channel phosphorylation/dephosphorylation mechanisms following activation of protein kinases or phosphatases. Modulation may also occur by the direct interaction of G-protein subunits, released in response to transmitter receptor activation, or of cellular metabolites such as Ca^{2+}, free fatty acids and nitric oxide (Table 8.2).

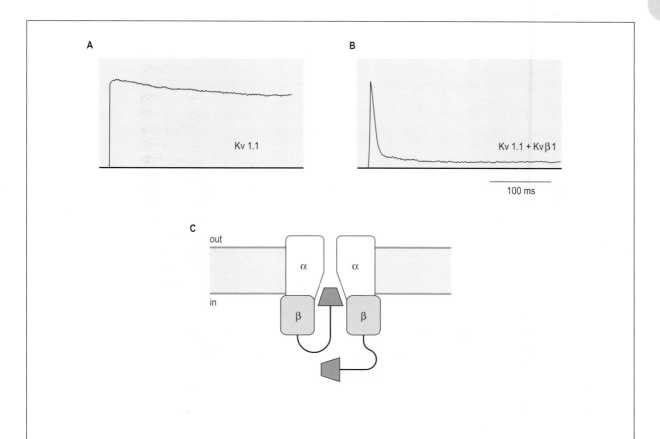

Fig. 8.8 K[+] current carried by the voltage-sensitive K[+] channel Kv1.1 when expressed alone (**A**) or together with the Kvβ1 subunit (**B**) which increases the rate of inactivation. It is proposed that the β1 subunit may provide a ball-and-chain inactivation mechanism. (Adapted from Rettig, J et al 1994 Nature 369: 289–294.)

Modulation	Channel	Modulator	Functional consequence	Tissue example
Phosphorylation	Voltage-gated Na[+]	cA-PK	Reduced P_O	Brain
		PKC	Reduced P_O, slowed inactivation	Brain
	Voltage-gated Ca[2+]	cA-PK	Increased P_O	Heart
		PKC	Increased or decreased P_O[a]	Heart
	Nicotinic ACh receptor	cA-PK	Increases the rate of desensitization	Skeletal muscle
G-protein	Voltage-gated Ca[2+]	G_O	Increased voltage-dependence for activation	Brain
	Voltage-gated Ca[2+]	G_s	Increased P_O	Heart
[Ca[2+]]	Voltage-gated Ca[2+]	Ca[2+]	Increases the rate of inactivation	Brain, heart, skeletal muscle
Free fatty acids	Voltage-gated K[+]	Free fatty acids	Increases activation	Smooth muscle
Nitric oxide	Ca[2+]-sensitive K[+]	NO	Increases activation	Smooth muscle
Neurotransmitters	NMDA receptor	Glycine	Increases P_O in response to glutamate	Brain

Table 8.2 Examples of channel modulation. [a] PKC produces an initial increase followed by a decrease in P_O.

Electrical conduction in nerves

The conduction velocity of an action potential over the surface of a nerve cell depends on the size of the cell and the electrical capacity of the cell membrane. The local circuit theory of propagation proposes that during an action potential the active region of membrane becomes more positively charged inside compared with adjacent regions and more negative outside compared with adjacent regions (see Fig. 8.5). Local currents are set up that raise the adjacent resting regions to threshold, resulting in the triggering of an action potential in those regions. Conduction velocity (Fig. 8.9) depends on:

- the size of the internal (axoplasmic) electrical resistance to local current flow, which is larger in smaller nerve fibres. Thus, conduction velocity is faster in larger nerve fibres
- the electrical capacitance of the cell membrane, i.e. the ability to store electric charge. A low membrane capacitance results in an increased conduction velocity as less work is required to depolarize adjacent regions of membrane to threshold for an action potential to be fired. In other words, conduction velocity is faster when the electrical resistance of the membrane is high.

Myelination

Myelinated nerves are formed from about four months of age by glial cells, which form a concentric wrapping of up to 200 layers thick around the nerve fibre to create a **myelin sheath** (Fig. 8.10). The cytoplasmic contents are withdrawn resulting in a multilayered membrane covering. Two types of glial cells are involved: **oligodendrocytes** in the central nervous system (CNS) and **Schwann** cells on peripheral nerves. The length of nerve wrapped by the myelin sheath of one glial cell is termed the **internode**. The unmyelinated regions between internodes are called **nodes of Ranvier**. Myelination reduces substantially the electrical capacitance of the internodal length such that electrical activity only occurs at the nodes of Ranvier. Thus, nerve impulse conduction occurs in a **saltatory** (jumping) manner, so increasing conduction velocity. In myelinated nerves the Na^+ channels that generate action potentials are located exclusively at the nodes of Ranvier. In some myelinated nerves, repolarization does not involve voltage-gated K^+ channels because the resting K^+ permeability is sufficient to restore the negative resting membrane potential.

If demyelination occurs, the excitation of successive nodes becomes progressively slowed as a result of the increased membrane capacitance, and conduction of the action potential ultimately fails. Insertion of new Na^+ channels in internodal regions of the membrane can restore some excitability after complete demyelination.

Multiple sclerosis

Multiple sclerosis is a disease of demyelination. Symptoms, such as loss of feeling, visual disturbance and muscle weakness, arise from dysfunctional sensory and motor neurone systems where fast axonal transmission is required.

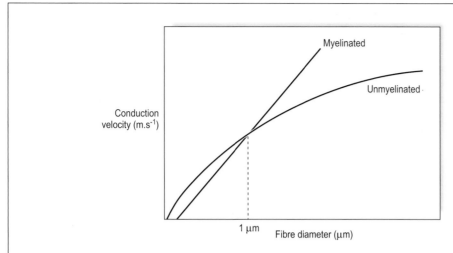

Fig. 8.9 Relationship between conduction velocity and nerve fibre diameter in myelinated and unmyelinated nerves. In unmyelinated fibres, the conduction velocity is proportional to √diameter, in myelinated nerves it is proportional to the diameter. Unmyelinated fibres have diameters less than 1 μm, and myelinated nerves greater than 1 μm. This ensures the maximum conduction velocity possible for a given nerve.

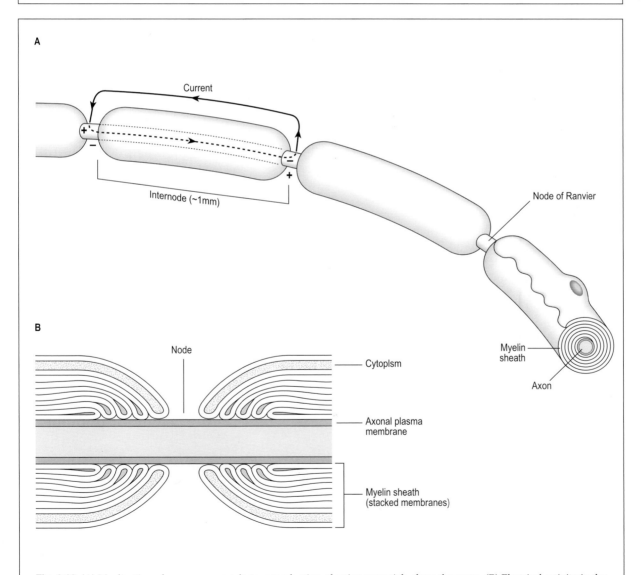

Fig. 8.10 (**A**) Myelination of nerves causes saltatory conduction of action potentials along the nerve. (**B**) Electrical activity in the nerve membrane occurs only at the nodes of Ranvier.

Cellular response to action potentials

Action potentials produce a biochemical response in the cell in which they are generated. By stimulating the opening of voltage-gated Ca^{2+} channels the action potential can produce a rise in free $[Ca^{2+}]_i$, which acts as an intracellular messenger to couple electrical excitation to cellular responses. For example, Ca^{2+} channels located specifically in presynaptic nerve terminals permit the gated entry of Ca^{2+} into the nerve terminal to act as a trigger for transmitter release. Ca^{2+}-induced release of Ca^{2+} from intracellular stores may also contribute to the rise in free $[Ca^{2+}]_i$ in response to an action potential.

Neurotransmission

Fast electrical transmission

As electrical activity in cells is generated on the plasma membrane, the passage of an electrical signal between cells can only occur when two cells are tightly physically coupled. This is accomplished by **gap junction channels**, which allow the passage of ions and small molecules between cells without leakage into the extracellular environment. Such junctions are found, for example, in heart muscle and some smooth muscles.

Chemical (synaptic) transmission

Chemical transmission of information between excitable cells occurs at specialized junctions called **synapses**. A chemical **transmitter** is released from the presynaptic structure of the signalling cell in response to depolarization and the influx of Ca^{2+}. The transmitter molecule diffuses across the synaptic cleft, binds to a specific receptor molecule on the postsynaptic cell and elicits a response in the postsynaptic cell (Fig. 8.11).

Neurotransmitter release

In nerve cells neurotransmitters are stored in, and released from, vesicular stores in the presynaptic nerve terminal. Release is, therefore, quantal in nature, each quantum representing the contents of one vesicle. In the unstimulated terminal, transmitter vesicles are held away from the plasma membrane by interaction with the actin cytoskeleton via synapsin and spectrin. Transmitter release occurs by exocytosis in response to raised $[Ca^{2+}]_i$ (Fig. 8.12). Ca^{2+} channels are localized very close to transmitter release sites on the presynaptic membrane. On excitation, the rise in $[Ca^{2+}]_i$ triggers several cellular events, which increase the probability of transmitter vesicle fusion with the plasma membrane. Ca^{2+}–stimulated depolymerization of the actin cytoskeleton and activation of Ca^{2+}–calmodulin-dependent protein kinase II (CaMII), which in turn phosphorylates and releases synapsin from the cytoskeleton, both result in increased mobility of the transmitter vesicles in the presynaptic nerve terminal. The increase in $[Ca^{2+}]$ also aids the docking of synaptic vesicles at the presynaptic membrane and may also facilitate the fusion process itself.

At the neuromuscular junction, approximately 0.25 ms (at 37°C) elapses between the arrival of the action potential and the release of transmitter (Fig. 8.13). This delay, together with the short time taken for the transmitter to diffuse across the synapse and activate postsynaptic receptors, constitutes the **synaptic delay** before the generation of a postsynaptic response. Note: released transmitter may bind to presynaptic receptors called autoreceptors to modulate the further release of transmitter (Fig. 8.12).

Microbial toxins acting on neurotransmission

Botulinum and tetanus toxins produce quite different clinical symptoms of parasympathetic and motor paralysis, and prolonged convulsions, respectively. Both toxins act presynaptically to cleave specific components of the SNARE ternary complexes, which target secretory vesicles to the synapse, thereby reducing transmitter release. Botulinum toxin inhibits acetylcholine release specifically while tetanus toxin reduces inhibitory amino acid transmitter release in the spinal cord. It is noteworthy that local injection of botulinum toxin can be used clinically to treat local muscle spasm.

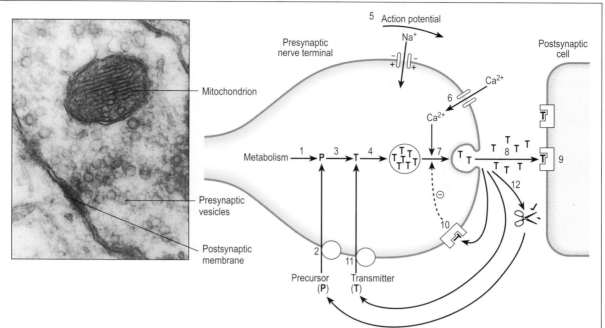

Fig. 8.11 Summary of the basic steps in chemical transmission. Each step represents a possible site of drug action. (1), Cellular metabolism; (2), precursor (P) uptake; (3), transmitter (T) synthesis; (4), sequestration of transmitter into vesicles; (5), depolarization of the presynaptic membrane by a propagated action potential; (6), Ca^{2+} entry through voltage-gated Ca^{2+} channels; (7), exocytosis and release of transmitter; (8), diffusion of transmitter across the synapse; (9), activation of postsynaptic receptors; (10), activation of presynaptic receptors (feedback modulation of transmitter release); (11), transmitter re-uptake; (12), chemical modification and inactivation of transmitter. (Adapted from Rang H P, Dale M M 1991 Pharmacology (2nd ed). Churchill Livingstone, Edinburgh, p139.) *Inset*: electron micrograph of an ultrathin section of a synapse. Bar = 250 nm. (EM courtesy of Professor Carole Hackney)

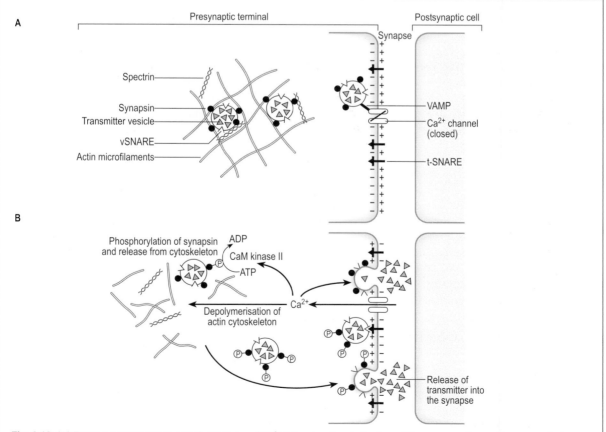

Fig. 8.12 (**A**) Resting presynaptic terminal. (**B**) Entry of Ca^{2+} following depolarization of the presynaptic membrane results in transmitter vesicle mobilization and fusion with the plasma membrane. VAMP, synaptobrevin; tSNARE, target membrane SNAP receptor; vSNARE, vescile SNAP receptor; CAMII, cellular adhesion molecule II.

Postsynaptic potentials

Chemical transmission can be fast or slow. The response in the cell may be excitatory or inhibitory (Table 8.3).

Fast synaptic neurotransmission

In **fast synaptic transmission**, the receptor comprises an integral ion channel (**ionotropic receptor**). Agonist binding to the receptor results in a change in conformation and opening of a gated channel (in the millisecond time range), which permits the flow of ions down their electrochemical gradient (see Chapter 6).

Excitatory neurotransmission

Excitatory transmitters open channels for ions with positive equilibrium potentials (Na^+, Ca^{2+}) or non-specific cation channels, resulting in membrane depolarization. The change in membrane protential caused by excitatory transmitters is called an **excitatory postsynaptic potential (EPSP)** (Fig. 8.14). Such potentials may bring the adjacent membrane containing voltage-gated channels to the threshold for action potential generation in the postsynaptic cell. For example, nicotinic acetylcholine receptor activation brings about a net influx of cations. The resulting rise in membrane potential is sufficient to trigger the opening of Na^+ channels in adjacent membrane areas to generate a full action potential.

At the neuromuscular junction small spontaneous postsynaptic potential changes of 0.5–1 mV can be observed under resting conditions. These **miniature endplate potentials (MEPPs)** result from the release from the presynaptic nerve terminal of a single vesicle (**quantum**) of acetylcholine and are too small to trigger an action potential in the muscle.

Neuromuscular blocking drugs in anaesthesia

Reflex movements in patients during surgery are commonly inhibited using two classes of drugs that block the action of acetylcholine:

- **Competitive antagonists** bind to nicotinic acetylcholine receptors in competition with acetylcholine and prevent channel opening, e.g. (+)-tubocurarine, gallamine and pancuronium.
- **Depolarizing blockers** act as agonists, initially opening the channel. The resulting membrane depolarization causes Na^+ channels to open and inactivate, producing a rapid 'phase I' block of neurotransmission. Over a period of time (minutes) the electrical excitability of the muscle membrane is restored as it repolarizes. However, neurotransmission remains blocked (phase II) as the continued presence of the blocker produces receptor desensitization (see Chapter 7), e.g. succinylcholine.

Inhibitory neurotransmission

Inhibitory transmitters open channels for ions with negative equilibrium potentials (K^+, Cl^-) resulting in membrane hyperpolarization and thereby reduced membrane excitability. The change in membrane potential caused by an inhibitory transmitter is called an **inhibitory postsynaptic potential (IPSP)** (Fig. 8.14). For example, glycine or GABA binding to glycine and $GABA_A$ receptors, respectively, open integral channels for Cl^- ions and bring about a membrane hyperpolarization.

Slow synaptic neurotransmission

In **slow synaptic transmission** the receptor (**metabotropic receptor**) signals to channel proteins via G-proteins within the membrane either directly (e.g. M_2-muscarinic acetylcholine receptor $\rightarrow G_i \rightarrow \beta\gamma \rightarrow K^+$ channel activation $\rightarrow$ M current) or indirectly via intracellular second messenger molecules (Fig. 8.15). Slow synaptic transmission occurs in the seconds to hours time range.

Termination of neurotransmission

Neurotransmission is terminated by removal of the transmitter from the synapse (see Fig. 8.11). This may be by degradation, e.g. cholinesterase in the synapse breaks down acetylcholine, or by reuptake into the presynaptic nerve terminal or an adjacent cell via specific transporters, e.g. noradrenaline.

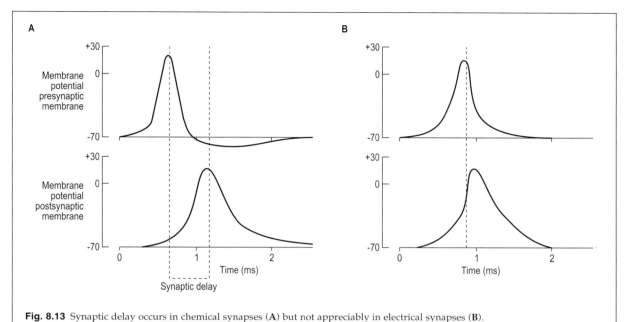

Fig. 8.13 Synaptic delay occurs in chemical synapses (**A**) but not appreciably in electrical synapses (**B**).

Transmission		Transmitter class	Transmitters
Fast	Excitatory	Amino acids	Glutamate, aspartate
		Amines	Acetylcholine (nicotinic), 5-HT
Slow	Inhibitory	Amino acids	Gamma aminobutyric acid, glycine
		Amines	Acetylcholine (muscarinic), dopamine, histamine, 5-HT, noradrenaline
		Peptides	Bradykinin, enkephalins, substance P

Table 8.3 Neurotransmitter systems. 5-HT, 5 hydroxytryptamine

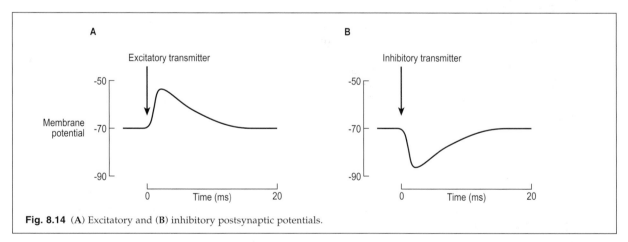

Fig. 8.14 (**A**) Excitatory and (**B**) inhibitory postsynaptic potentials.

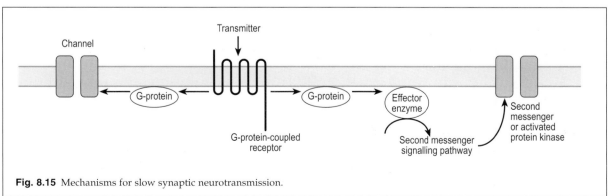

Fig. 8.15 Mechanisms for slow synaptic neurotransmission.

Examples of the integration of signalling mechanisms in cellular processes

Glucose-stimulated insulin release

Glucose-stimulated insulin release from β cells of the pancreatic islets of Langerhans depends on the coupling of metabolism to the modification of ion channel activity (Fig. 8.16). Glucose uptake is proportional to circulating glucose concentrations because of the high K_M of the GLUT2 transporter. The internalized glucose is then metabolized rapidly with the concomitant production of ATP. In the resting β cell, active ATP-sensitive K^+ (K_{ATP}) channels contribute to the resting membrane potential. These channels close in response to raised ATP concentration and probably also falling ADP concentration. This results in a gradual membrane depolarization and activation of L-type, voltage-gated Ca^{2+} channels. The resultant Ca^{2+} influx raises $[Ca^{2+}]_i$ and triggers the exocytosis of insulin-containing secretory vesicles. In addition to the repolarizing influence of activated delayed rectifier K^+ channels, the raised $[Ca^{2+}]_i$ also stimulates the opening of Ca^{2+}-sensitive K^+ channels that contribute to the repolarization of the membrane.

Although not direct stimulators of insulin secretion, hormones such as glucagon (signalling metabolic stress) and glucagon-like peptide 1 (GLP-1, signalling arrival of a food bolus in the gut) potentiate glucose-stimulated insulin secretion. Signalling by these hormones is via cyclic AMP and the activation of cA-PK. Resulting phosphorylation of ion channels and other mechanisms involved in stimulus-secretion coupling increase the response to a given concentration of glucose. These hormones do not stimulate insulin secretion alone as they require Ca^{2+}–calmodulin complex formation for the activation of cA-PK.

Ion channel modulation in the treatment of non-insulin-dependent diabetes mellitus

Sulphonylurea K_{ATP} channel blockers, e.g. glibenclamide, will also trigger insulin release by producing a membrane depolarization. This class of drugs is used in patients with mild non-insulin-dependent (type II) diabetes mellitus to overcome their hyperglycaemia and insulin resistance by raising endogenous insulin secretion.

Visual transduction

In the retina (rods and cones), it is the breakdown rather than synthesis of cyclic GMP that transmits information concerning photon detection (Fig. 8.17). In the dark, levels of cyclic GMP are maintained at a relatively raised level, which acts on cyclic GMP-operated ion channels to allow Na^+ and Ca^{2+} to enter the cell to depolarize the membrane. Photons of light are detected by a photosensitive prosthetic (helper) group, 11-cis-retinal, located in the ligand-binding cleft of the G-protein-coupled receptor opsin, which together form rhodopsin. The resulting conformational change in rhodopsin is transduced into a cellular event by the specific G-protein, transducin (Gt). Gtα-GTP activates cyclic GMP phosphodiesterase leading to a reduction in cyclic GMP concentration and, thereby, Na^+ conductance. As a result, the membrane becomes more polarized and transmitter release, which forms the signalling output to the CNS, is reduced.

Excitotoxicity

The release of high concentrations of excitatory amino acid transmitters, e.g. glutamate, in the brain is a major factor in cerebral damage after ischaemia (reduced blood supply) in head injury and degenerative brain diseases such as epilepsy and Huntington's chorea. The glutamate stimulates a Ca^{2+} overload in neurones by several reinforcing mechanisms, which lead to a release of further glutamate and, ultimately, cell death (Fig. 8.18). Cell death in response to Ca^{2+} may involve the activation of intracellular proteases and lipases, the impairment of mitochondrial function and the generation of free radicals. In view of these excitotoxic mechanisms there is considerable interest in the possible use of NMDA and Ca^{2+} channel antagonists in the treatment of head injury, epilepsy and stroke.

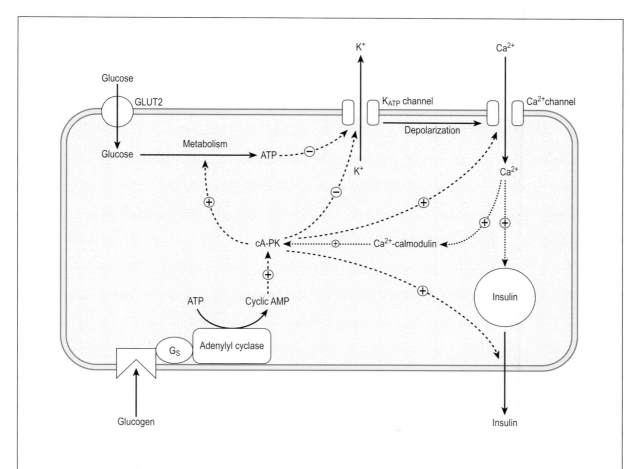

Fig. 8.16 Stimulus-secretion coupling in pancreatic β cells. Glucagon potentiates glucose-stimulated insulin release but is unable to stimulate insulin release alone. GLUT2, glucose transporter 2; cA-PK, cyclic AMP-dependent protein kinase.

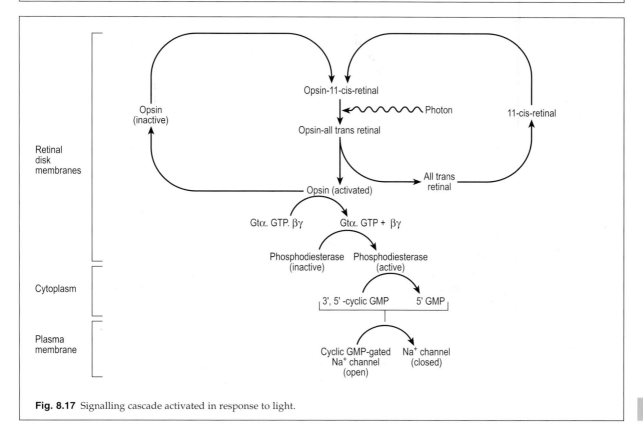

Fig. 8.17 Signalling cascade activated in response to light.

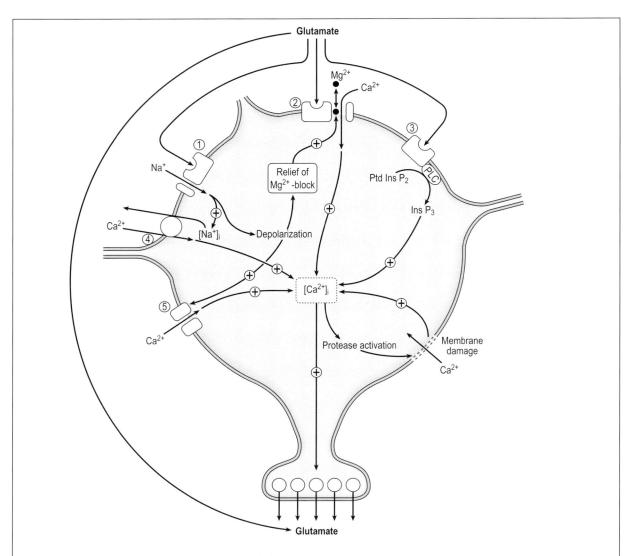

Fig. 8.18 Proposed mechanisms of glutamate excitotoxicity. (1) Na⁺ entry and membrane depolarization on glutamate activation of the AMPA/kainate glutamate receptor. (2) The NMDA receptor is blocked by Mg^{2+} at resting membrane potentials. Membrane depolarization relieves the block and permits glutamate-stimulated entry of Ca^{2+} ions. (3) Activation of metabotropic glutamate receptors stimulates $PtdInsP_2$ phospholipase C (PLC) activity and hence the formation of $InsP_3$ and the release of internal Ca^{2+} stores. (4) Membrane depolarization and raised $[Na^+]_i$ cause the Na⁺–Ca²⁺ exchanger to operate in reverse mode contributing to Ca^{2+} influx. (5) Membrane depolarization activates voltage-operated Ca^{2+} channels. Raised $[Ca^{2+}]_i$ stimulates further release of glutamate and stimulates cytotoxic protease activity. (Adapted from Rang H P, Dale M M 1991 Pharmacology (2nd ed). Churchill Livingstone, Edinburgh, p598.)

Further reading

Aidley D J 1990 The physiology of excitable cells, 3rd edn. Cambridge University Press, Cambridge

Aidley D J, Stanfield P R 1996 Ion channels: molecules in action. Cambridge University Press, Cambridge

Ghosh A, Greenberg M E 1995 Calcium signaling in neurons – molecular mechanisms and cellular consequences. Science 268: 239–247

Hoffman E P, Lehmannhorn F, Rudel R 1995 Overexcited or inactive – ion channels in muscle disease. Cell 80: 681–686

Holz G G, Habener J F 1992 Signal transduction crosstalk in the endocrine system: pancreatic β-cells and the glucose competence concept. Trends in Biochemical Sciences 17: 388–393

Kumar N M, Gilula N B 1996 The gap junction communication channel. Cell 84: 381–388

Lehman-Horn F, Rudel R 1996 Molecular pathophysiology of voltage-gated ion channels. Reviews of Physiology, Biochemistry and Pharmacology 128: 195–268

Sudhof T C 1995 The synaptic vesicle cycle – a cascade of protein–protein interactions. Nature 375: 645–653

Revision questions

1. What is the major mechanism for the maintenance of the resting membrane potential in cells?

2. Using the Nernst equation calculate the K^+ equilibrium potential (E_K) at 37°C for cells with the intra- and extracellular fluid ion compositions as given in Table 8.1 is –95 mV. Explain why the measured resting membrane potential is often more positive than this value.

3. The plasma K^+ concentration in a hyperkalaemic patient was found to be 7.5 mM. Assuming a similar value for the interstitial fluid, what would be the consequences for the K^+ equilibrium potential (E_K) of peripheral cells? (use the Nernst equation). What would be the clinical consequences of a raised K^+ concentration in this patient?

4. Outline the ionic basis of the action potential in nerve fibres.

5. Nerve fibres become refractory to further action potentials just after the firing of an action potential. Why does this occur?

6. Compare and contrast the structures of the pore-forming subunits of voltage-gated and voltage-insensitive cation channels.

7. What is saltatory conduction in nerve fibres? Why does it occur? How does saltatory conduction influence conduction velocity in nerve fibres?

8. Draw an annotated diagram of a synapse to illustrate the important processes necessary for neurotransmission. How is neurotransmitter release stimulated? How does the neurotransmitter exert an effect on the postsynaptic cell? How is neurotransmission terminated?

9. Describe excitatory postsynaptic potentials and inhibitory postsynaptic potentials. Outline how each is generated.

10. What mechanisms underlie fast and slow neurotransmission?

11. How does glucose stimulate the release of insulin from pancreatic β cells?

12. How is light detected and converted into an electrical signal in the retina?

Answers to revision questions

1. The main influence on resting membrane potential is the efflux of K^+ through K^+ channels.

2. Resting membrane potential is usually greater than E_K owing to a low level of inward leak of Na^+ and Ca^{2+} ions.

3. The calculated E_K is –81 mV. The resting membrane potential will be less polarized than in a normal individual and, hence, excitable membranes will be more readily depolarized. Greater excitability in the heart will lead to ventricular arrhythmia and possibly ventricular fibrillation. Treatment of the hyperkalaemia is, therefore, most important.

4. The rapid depolarizing phase of the action potential results from the influx of Na^+ ions through voltage-gated Na^+ channels. Rapid inactivation of opened Na^+ channels together with efflux of K^+ through slow opening of delayed rectifier K^+ channels contribute to the later repolarization phase. A period of hyperpolarization at the end of the action potential occurs because of continued K^+ influx as a consequence of the slow inactivation of the K_{DR} channels.

5. The refractory period in nerve fibres after the firing of an action potential is due to the inactivation of Na^+ channels. This renders the membrane inexcitable until the channels have been 'reprimed' upon membrane polarization.

6. In both channel types the pore is formed by four hairpin loops (SS1–SS2) folded into the membrane from the extracellular side of the membrane, each supported by two transmembrane α-helices. An additional four transmembrane segments are present at the N-terminal of the voltage-gated channels. Of particular importance is the S4 segment, which, by virtue of its content of positively charged residues, constitutes the voltage-sensor of these channels.

7. Saltatory conduction occurs where electrical excitation jumps between nodes of Ranvier in myelinated nerves, rather than propagating along the whole fibre in unmyelinated nerves. It occurs as a result of myelination of the nerve fibre, which reduces the capacitance of the nerve in that region and the localization of channels at the nodes of Ranvier, both of which preclude electrical activity in the internodal regions. Saltatory conduction increases conduction velocity in nerve fibres.

8. See Fig. 8.12. Transmitter release is stimulated in response to the arrival of an action potential on the presynaptic membrane. Neurotransmitter release is stimulated by the entry of Ca^{2+} through voltage-sensitive Ca^{2+} channels that open in response to the arrival of an action potential in the presynaptic membrane. Neurotransmitters bind to specific receptors on the postsynaptic membrane to elicit a response. Neurotransmission may be terminated by degradation of the neurotransmitter in the synapse, e.g. acetylcholine, or by reuptake into the presynaptic terminal or adjacent cells, e.g. noradrenaline.

9. EPSPs and IPSPs are depolarizing and hyperpolarizing currents, respectively. Both are generated in response to the opening of ligand-gated ion channels. EPSPs are carried by ions with positive equilibrium potentials (Na^+, Ca^{2+}), e.g. in response to transmitters such as acetylcholine and glutamate. IPSPs are generated as a result of the opening of Cl^- channels in response to transmitters such as GABA and glycine.

10. Fast neurotransmission is mediated by the rapid opening of ligand-gated ion channels. Slow neurotransmission is mediated by receptors without integral ion channel activity that stimulate channel opening either via a direct interaction with G-proteins or indirectly following stimulation of an intracellular signalling pathway.

11. Metabolism of glucose results in the production of ATP. The rise in ATP concentration inhibits K_{ATP} channels which contribute to the resting membrane potential, thereby causing a membrane depolarization. Voltage-gated Ca^{2+} channels open in response to this depolarization admitting Ca^{2+} necessary to stimulate the release of vesicular stores of insulin.

12. A photon provides the energy for the conversion of 11-cis-retinal to all trans-retinal within the light-sensing rhodopsin molecule. A resulting conformational change is transmitted to transducin, which dissociates to release $G_t\alpha$-GTP. This activates cyclic GMP phosphodiesterase to reduce the cellular concentration of cyclic GMP, which in turn reduces the activity of cyclic GMP-gated Na^+ channels. The resultant membrane polarization reduces transmitter release and so reduces the signalling output to the brain.

The cytoskeleton and muscle contraction

In eukaryotes, the cytoskeleton is a complex framework of structural protein filaments that defines the shape of a cell. It is a dynamic structure, and is responsible for changes in cell shape and cell movement. It also contributes to the movement of intracellular organelles and other cytoplasmic components and is, therefore, important in organization and microcompartmentalization within the cell. In contractile muscle cells the cytoskeleton is further modified to provide the contractile machinery.

The cytoskeleton

Attachment sites

Cellular cytoskeletons can make attachments that link them to the extracellular matrix. Several specialized junctional complexes have been partially characterized that link particular cytoskeletal structures to specific extracellular structures (Table 9.1). In each case the connection is made by a transmembranous protein that interacts with components on both sides of the membrane (see Chapter 10). At the intracellular surface of the membrane, cytoskeletal elements are attached to the transmembrane proteins by accessory proteins such as α-actinin, talin and vinculin. The junctional structures are highly complex and sensitive to phosphorylation at multiple sites. Therefore, intracellular signalling pathways can impinge on cytoskeletal activity through these structures.

Filamentous structures in cytoskeletons

The cytoskeletons of all cells are based on three basic filamentous structures – **microfilaments** (7 nm diameter), **microtubules** (24 nm diameter) and **intermediate filaments** (10 nm diameter) – in which actin, tubulin and intermediate filament proteins form the core structure, respectively. Depending on the cell type, cytoskeletons may be composed of just one filamentous element or a combination of two or three of the basic structures. In addition, a large number of **accessory proteins** can be involved. These confer the cell-specific and dynamic properties to the cytoskeleton. Accessory proteins can influence the position of the cytoskeleton within the cell by controlling the length of the filamentous structures and their association with other protein complexes, organelles, membranes and the extracellular matrix. In addition, they can permit modification of the cytoskeleton in response to intracellular metabolic changes and intracellular signalling pathways, in particular changes in $[Ca^{2+}]_i$.

Each of the core structural proteins forms helical filaments, which have a polarity due to chemically distinct heads and tails. Each protein exists in multiple isoforms, some of which are tissue specific.

Microfilaments

The major constituent of microfilaments is the globular protein actin, which is a component of all eukaryotic cells. The actin monomer (G-actin) possesses sites for divalent cations and nucleotides and binds Mg^{2+} and ATP. Monomers can associate to form dimers and trimers, and trimers are sufficiently stable to form nucleation centres for the further polymerization into actin filaments (F-actin). Actin filaments consist of two strings of monomers in a right-handed helical structure which achieves one turn every 14 actin monomers (Fig. 9.2). Each actin monomer has a polarity and monomers associate head to tail. Polarity of the growing microfilament can be defined by the association of heavy meromyosin (a proteolytic fragment of the actin-binding protein myosin containing the two globular myosin heads, see below), which forms an arrowhead pattern on the filament and the poles of the microfilament can be designated as the pointed (–) and barbed (+) ends. Elongation can occur at both ends but is usually faster at the barbed (+) end. G-actin contains either bound ATP or ADP. The rate of binding of G-actin-ATP to growing microfilaments is much faster and binding is followed by rapid ATP hydrolysis, although this is not essential to polymerization. ATP hydrolysis allows a microfilament to treadmill, i.e. G-actin-ATP monomers are added at one end while G-actin-ADP dissociates from the other (Fig. 9.3). Growing microfilaments can also break, generating new free ends. These can behave as nuclei for further polymerization or may anneal with a second microfilament.

Junctional structure	Functional interaction	Cytoskeleton
Adherens junctions (zona adherens)	Cell–cell	Actin filaments
Desmosomes (macula adherens)	Cell–cell	Intermediate filaments
Focal adhesions	Cell–substrate	Actin filaments and stress fibres
Hemidesmosomes	Cell–substrate	Intermediate filaments
Erythroid cytoskeleton	Membrane attachment	Spectrin–actin network
Striated muscle	Membrane attachment	Actin filaments

Table 9.1 Cytoskeletal attachments to junctional complexes

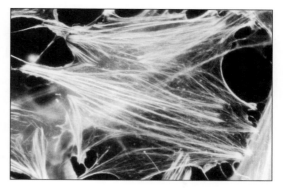

Fig. 9.1 Micrograph of fibroblasts stained with immunofluorescent marker to reveal stress fibres in the actin cytoskeleton. (Courtesy of Dr Jim Norman)

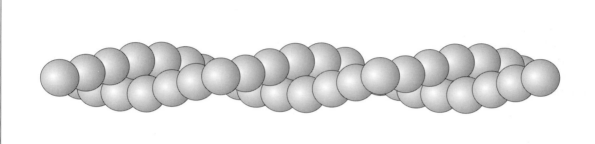

Fig. 9.2 Actin microfilaments consist of a right-handed double stranded helix of polymerized actin molecules.

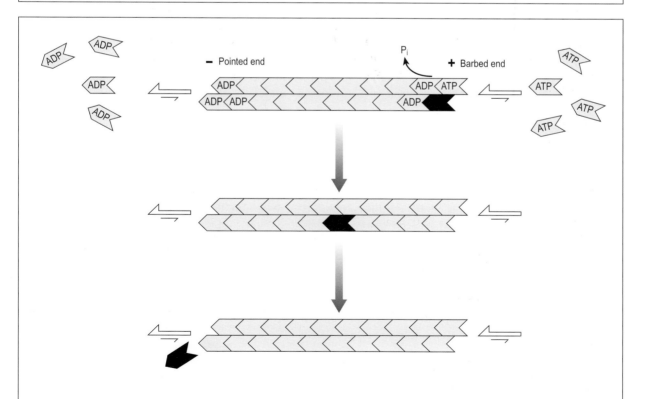

Fig. 9.3 Treadmilling in actin microfilaments illustrated by the passage of the shaded actin molecule through the filament. Capping of microfilament ends with accessory proteins can prevent treadmilling

Microtubules

Microtubules, like microfilaments, are formed from linear polymers composed of **tubulin** subunits (Fig. 9.4). The tubulins are amongst the most highly conserved proteins known. Unlike G-actin, however, the tubulin subunit is an αβ dimer. Both α- and β-tubulin can bind GTP and GDP but only the β subunit can exchange its bound nucleotide with GTP in the cytoplasm when in the dimeric subunit form. Tubulin polymerization shares many similarities with actin polymerization. Subunits must first associate to form a nucleus, upon which bidirectional polymerization of a polar microtubule continues. This is associated with hydrolysis of bound GTP, which again, although not necessary to the polymerization process, permits treadmilling of the tubulin polymer in vitro. In cells, however, the slow growing (–) end is capped by its association with the **centrosome complex**, preventing treadmilling. Microtubules are dynamic structures and rapid depolymerization and repolymerization is a characteristic of their function. New tubulin dimers can be added to rapidly growing protofilaments as long as the terminal tubulin molecule is in the GTP-bound form. If hydrolysis of GTP to GDP occurs in the terminal tubulin, dissociation is favoured and the filament breaks down. Also, as in actin microfilaments, breakage and annealing of tubulin polymers allows for changes in the number and density of microtubule ends without any change in subunit number. Tubulin polymerization is inhibited by raised $[Ca^{2+}]_i$ and low temperature.

Tubulin-binding drugs are used in cancer therapy

Colchicine, nocodazole, taxol and vinblastine all bind to tubulin and interfere with normal tubulin dynamics. Because microtubules are involved in spindle formation in cell division, these pharmaceutical agents are often used as antimitotic drugs in cancer chemotherapy. Colchicine is also used to treat diseases of cell infiltration. In gout it is used to prevent the migration of neutrophils into joints and it is also used in dermatological diseases that involve leucocyte infiltration, e.g. psoriasis.

Microtubules are hollow cylinders of 24 nm in diameter and consist of 13 protofilaments of tubulin subunits (Fig. 9.4). Tubulin subunits are added to the protofilaments such that α and β tubulins alternate giving the protofilament and the microtubule polarity. Microtubules do not form in the cytoplasm in the absense of nucleating **centrosome complexes** as the rate of dissociation from the slow-growing end is too fast. The centrosome complex caps this end of the microtubule, thus permitting polymerization. Centrosomes are composed of a pair of **centrioles** at right angles to each other, each composed of tubules of nine, short triplet microtubules (Fig. 9.5), surrounded by **pericentriolar material** to which the microtubules are attached.

Intermediate filaments

Intermediate filaments are a family of cytoplasmic filamentous structures that are intermediate in diameter (10 nm) between microfilaments and microtubules. This group of proteins is much more heterogeneous than the actins and tubulins, and each type of filament is composed of a distinct protein or proteins (Table 9.2). Unlike actin and tubulin, which are globular proteins, the intermediate filament proteins are fibrous. Each intermediate filament protein has an homologous α-helical core structure of 310 amino acids (with three non-helical gaps) with subunit-specific N- and C-termini of variable length. Filaments are initiated by the formation of a parallel, coiled-coil structure composed of the homologous core structure of two subunits. Intermediate filaments are formed by polymerization of these dimeric structures (Fig. 9.6). Because the intermediate filament structure is based on the homologous core structure, co-polymerization of mixed oligomers is possible when certain subunits are co-expressed in the same tissue (see Table 9.2). Not all subunit combinations are stable. Where co-expression of incompatible subunits occurs, homo-oligomers of each protein are formed, e.g. keratins and vimentin in epithelial cells.

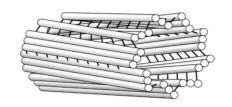
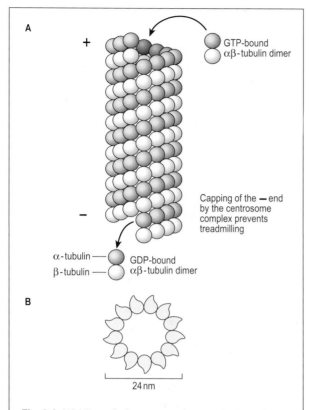

A

+

GTP-bound
αβ-tubulin dimer

Capping of the — end
by the centrosome
complex prevents
treadmilling

−

α-tubulin
β-tubulin

GDP-bound
αβ-tubulin dimer

B

24 nm

Fig. 9.4 (**A**) Microtubule structure showing the helical array of αβ tubulin dimers and treadmilling. (**B**) Transverse section of a microtubule.

Fig. 9.5 Schematic diagram of a centriole. Two centrioles orientated perpendicular to each other form nucleation sites for microtubular cytoskeletal structures.

Intermediate filament	Subunits (M_r)	Cell type
Keratin	Type I acidic keratins	Epithelial cells
	Type II neutral/basic keratins	
Neurofilaments	NF_L	Neurons
	NF_M	
	NF_H	
Nuclear lamina	Lamins A, B and C	All nucleated cells
Vimentin-containing	Vimentin	Fibroblasts
	Vimentin + desmin	Muscle cells
	Vimentin + glial fibrillary acidic protein	Glial cells

Table 9.2 Intermediate filaments.
Note: detection of cell specific expression of intermediate filament protein combinations using intermediate filament specific monoclonal antibodies has provided a useful method for determining the origin of metastatic cancer cells.

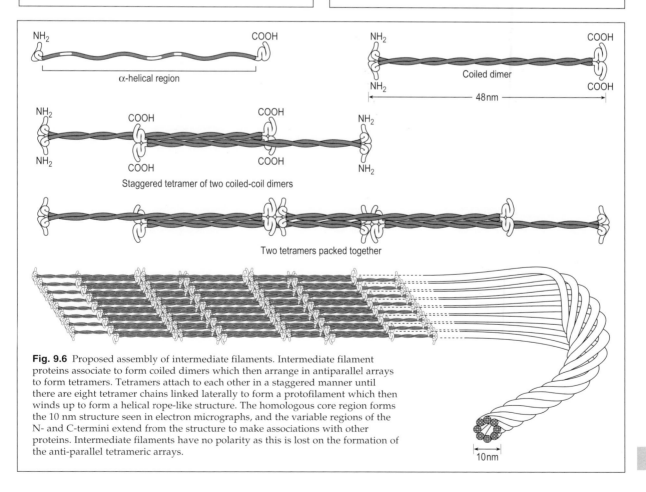

NH₂

COOH

α-helical region

NH₂

COOH

Coiled dimer

NH₂

COOH

48nm

NH₂

COOH

COOH

NH₂

NH₂

COOH

COOH

NH₂

Staggered tetramer of two coiled-coil dimers

Two tetramers packed together

10nm

Fig. 9.6 Proposed assembly of intermediate filaments. Intermediate filament proteins associate to form coiled dimers which then arrange in antiparallel arrays to form tetramers. Tetramers attach to each other in a staggered manner until there are eight tetramer chains linked laterally to form a protofilament which then winds up to form a helical rope-like structure. The homologous core region forms the 10 nm structure seen in electron micrographs, and the variable regions of the N- and C-termini extend from the structure to make associations with other proteins. Intermediate filaments have no polarity as this is lost on the formation of the anti-parallel tetrameric arrays.

Accessory proteins

The properties of microfilaments and microtubules can be further modified by a large number of accessory proteins that interact with them. A wide range of proteins interact with actin microfilaments (Table 9.3). Two major classes of **microtubule-associated proteins** (**MAPs**) have been identified that play roles in microtubule assembly, crosslinking, stabilization and transport: a small group of high molecular weight MAPs (200–300 kDa) and a group of low molecular weight or tau MAPs (40–60 kDa).

Spectrin–actin cytoskeleton of the erythrocyte

The best understood cytoskeleton is the spectrin–actin cytoskeleton of erythrocytes, which confers the biconcave shape to these cells. The erythrocyte cytoskeleton is based on the peripheral membrane protein **spectrin**, which is a long, floppy, rod-like molecule consisting of a dimer of large α and β subunits (Fig. 9.7). The α and β subunits wind together to form an antiparallel heterodimer and two heterodimers then form a head-to-head association to form a heterotetramer of $\alpha_2\beta_2$. These heterotetrameric rods are crosslinked into networks by short actin protofilaments (~14 actin monomers), which associate towards the ends of the spectrin heterotetramers (Fig. 9.8). This interaction is stabilized by a protein called **band 4.1** (after its relative migration in SDS-PAGE) and **adducin**. The spectrin–actin network is attached to the plasma membrane through accessory proteins that link spectrin to integral membrane proteins. **Ankyrin** (band 4.9) forms a link between the spectrin and the **anion exchange protein** (band 3), and band 4.1 forms an association with **glycophorin A**. Attachment of integral membrane proteins to the cytoskeleton restricts the lateral mobility of these membrane proteins.

Haemolytic anaemias

The erythrocyte cytoskeleton is a very important structure in maintaining the deformability necessary for erythrocytes to make their passage through capillary beds without lysis. In the common dominant form of **hereditary spherocytosis**, spectrin levels may be depleted by 40–50%. The cells round up and become much less resistant to lysis during passage through the capillaries and are cleared by the spleen. The shortened in vivo survival of red blood cells and the inability of the bone marrow to compensate for their reduced life-span leads to **haemolytic anaemia**. Other forms of hereditary spherocytosis also exist where mutated cytoskeletal elements with dysfunctional binding sites for other components are expressed. Similarly, in **hereditary elliptocytosis**, a common defect is a spectrin molecule that is unable to form heterotetramers, resulting in fragile elliptoid cells. Even simple treatment with cytochalasin drugs, which cap the growing end of polymerizing actin filaments, can alter the deformability of the erythrocyte.

Cytoskeleton and blood pressure

Mutations in the cytoskeletal linker protein adducin have been shown to be associated genetically with essential hypertension. These mutants modify membrane ion transport in ways similar to perturbations seen in hypertensive patients. It may be that cytoskeletal perturbation resulting in altered ion homeostasis in vascular tissues may be responsible for the development of hypertension in some patients.

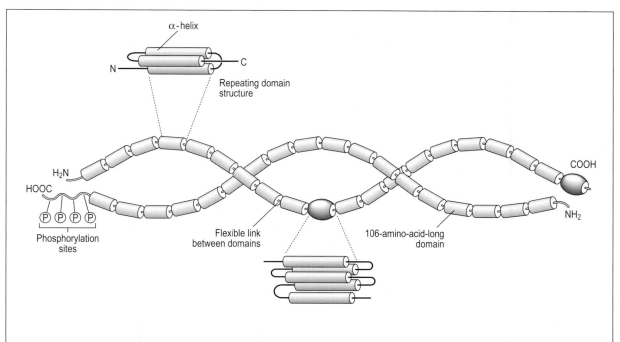

Fig. 9.7 Schematic diagram of a spectrin molecule composed of an antiparallel array of α and β subunits coiled together.

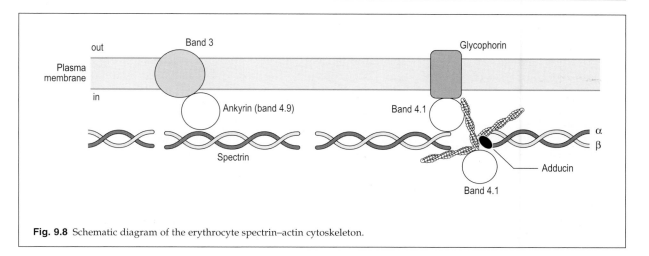

Fig. 9.8 Schematic diagram of the erythrocyte spectrin–actin cytoskeleton.

Protein	Function
α-Actinin	Filament attachment and bundling
Cap Z	Caps (+) ends of filaments
Filamin/fodrin	Crosslinks filaments (spectrin-like)
Fimbrin	Filament bundling — cross-bridges adjacent microfilaments
Gelosin/severin	Cuts actin filaments into protofilaments
Myosin I	Vesicle transport on filaments
Myosin II	Sliding filaments in muscles
Profilin	Binds G-actin, prevents polymerization
Spectrin	Crosslinks filaments into cytoskeletal network
Tropomyosin	Filament stabilization/regulates binding of myosin
Villin	Filament bundling (low $[Ca^{2+}]_i$)
	Cleaves actin filaments (μM $[Ca^{2+}]_i$)

Table 9.3 Actin-binding proteins

Spectrin supergene family

Spectrin or spectrin-like molecules are found in non-erythroid tissues where they contribute to cytoskeletal structures close to the plasma membrane but also as multifunctional crosslinkers within the cytoplasm. α-Spectrin may associate with an alternatively spliced erythroid β subunit or with a non-erythroid β spectrin, to produce **fodrin** (spectrin II).

Two other proteins with spectrin-like repeating structures of three α-helices and conserved N-terminal domains are **α-actinin** and **dystrophin**. The similarity of these proteins to spectrin suggests that they have all descended from a common ancestral gene. α-Actinin is an actin-bundling protein (c.f. Z discs) and dystrophin is proposed to attach actin filaments to the plasma membrane in skeletal muscle. The absence of dystrophin in Duchenne muscular dystrophy (DMD) underlies the muscle weakness in this disease (see Chapter 10).

Skeletal muscle

Microfilamentous structure of skeletal muscle

Shortening in muscle cells is mediated by the progressive overlap of interdigitated thick and thin filaments composed predominantly of myosin and actin, respectively.

Thick filaments

The core of thick filaments is composed of myosin. Myosin molecules are composed of two identical heavy chains and two pairs of light chains, one of each per head (Fig. 9.9). The α-helical, C-terminal domains of the two myosin heavy chains form a coiled-coil, resulting in a long, rigid, rod-like structure. The N-terminal head regions provide sites for interaction with two light chains each, a site for interaction with polymerized actin filaments and a catalytic ATPase domain. The hydrolysis of ATP by myosin provides the free energy necessary to drive the contractile process.

Thick filaments are formed by the tail-to-tail association of myosin molecules to form insoluble, rod-like complexes of between 300 and 400 molecules. The structure is stabilized by interactions between the myosin tail rods, which form a six-fold axis of symmetry. The head groups protrude to the outside of the structure at both ends leaving a central bare zone. The 60° separation between head groups, determined by the symmetry of myosin molecules in the thick filament, places the head groups in alignment with adjacent actin filaments in the structure of the contractile element, the **sarcomere**.

Thin filaments

Thin filaments are composed of actin microfilaments and two accessory proteins, **tropomyosin** and **troponin**. Unlike cytoskeletal actin microfilaments, which undergo repeated polymerization and depolymerization in response to cellular shape changes, microfilaments that form part of the contractile machinery are stable structures.

Tropomyosin is a long rod-like molecule composed predominantly of α-helix. In thin filaments, tropomyosin molecules form head-to-tail, coiled-coil dimers and lie either along the surface or along the groove of the F-actin helical structure (Fig. 9.10). When positioned on the surface, in resting muscle, tropomyosin blocks the interaction with the thick myosin filaments, whereas movement to the groove region, in response to raised $[Ca^{2+}]_i$, reveals the myosin binding site and permits activity of the contractile machinery. Ca^{2+} is, therefore, the trigger for and facilitator of muscle contraction by controlling the allosteric inhibition of thin and thick filament interaction by tropomyosin. Ca^{2+} sensitivity is conferred by the troponin.

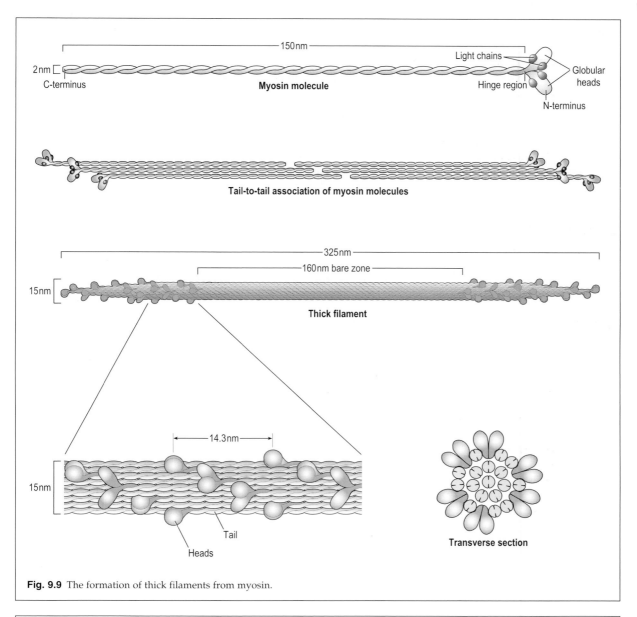

Fig. 9.9 The formation of thick filaments from myosin.

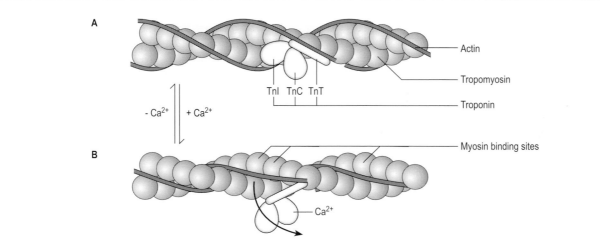

Fig. 9.10 Model of Ca^{2+}-stimulated movements of troponin and tropomyosin to reveal myosin binding sites on actin microfilaments. Ca^{2+} binding to the troponin TnC subunit induces a conformational change in the globular TnC–TnI domain causing it to move away from the actin filament. This movement removes the inhibition on tropomyosin movement into the filament groove.

The sarcomere

Under the light microscope vertebrate muscle has a striated appearance. Skeletal muscle is made up of bundles of parallel cells and each multinucleated cell contains bundles of myofibrils. When these are observed for relaxed muscle under the electron microscope, a repeating structure (2.4 μm) of the functional contractile element, the sarcomere, becomes apparent. An alternating pattern of light (**I band**, isotropic) and dark (**A band**, anisotropic) bands is observed (Fig. 9.11). A dark line bisecting the I band is the **Z band** or **Z disc** and the segment of myofibril between two Z discs, containing an A band and two half I bands, is defined as a **sarcomere**. Thin filaments are attached to Z discs and constitute the light half I band and the darker region of the A band at each end of the sacomere. Association of the growing (barbed, +) ends of actin microfilaments to α-**actinin** of the Z disc is through **cap Z protein**. This interaction probably serves to prevent further polymerization or depolymerization of the microfilaments. The A band represents the distribution of myosin thick filaments and the lighter **H band** at the centre represents the myosin tail region of the thick filaments, which are not overlapping with thin filaments. The dark **M line**, which bisects the H band, is a region of crosslinking between thick filaments where the polarity of the thick filament is reversed. Cross-sectional views at various points along the sarcomere reveal a triagonal array for the thick filaments and a hexagonal array for the thin filaments. This structure is stabilized by two further proteins with elastic properties, which are both attached to the Z disc: titin extends and attaches to myosin thick filaments and nebulin lies alongside actin microfilaments.

On muscle contraction the distance between Z discs is reduced (from 2.4 μm to ~1.6 μm) as is the length of the I band. The length of the A band remains unchanged. This important observation formed the basis of the 'sliding filament' model of muscle contraction.

Muscle contraction

The sliding filament model of muscle contraction: role of ATP

The opposite movement of thick and thin filaments during contraction is achieved by a cyclic interaction between actin and myosin of attachment, pulling and detachment. The proposed mechanism involves a large change in position of the head group of the myosin molecule while attached to actin to drive the opposite movement of the two filaments (Fig. 9.12). In resting muscle, tropomyosin prevents molecular association between actin and myosin. On stimulation this constraint is removed and the contractile cycle is initiated by the interaction of actin and myosin head groups containing ADP and P_i in their catalytic site. On binding actin, P_i is released from the myosin head group, which in response undergoes a large rotation in the 'hinge' region of the molecule between the head group and tail. This large conformational change, known as the 'power stroke', pulls the myosin molecule along the actin filament by approximately 7.5 nm. At the end of the power stroke, ADP is released from the myosin active site and is replaced by ATP. This leads to a rapid dissociation of the myosin heads from actin and reversal of the conformational change of the head group. Hydrolysis of the bound ATP returns the myosin head group to the high-energy, myosin–ADP–P_i form, priming it for a further round of the cycle. The myosin head groups in thick filaments do not move in synchrony but rather can be found at different phases at any one moment. This ensures that the overall contractile process is smooth.

The presence of actin can increase the rate of ATP hydrolysis by myosin 100-fold, but it is noteworthy that the free-energy-releasing step occurs after the ATP-hydrolysis step. Thus, the free energy from ATP hydrolysis is passed on indirectly to the power stroke through the high-energy conformation of the myosin–ADP–P_i intermediate. Although not part of the active site, the myosin light chains can also modulate the rate of ATP hydrolysis and the particular isoforms expressed in any muscle can determine the twitch speed of the muscle.

Rigor mortis

In the absence of ATP the actin–myosin interaction at the end of the power stroke remains associated in the so-called rigor complex. This is the process of rigor mortis in dead muscle.

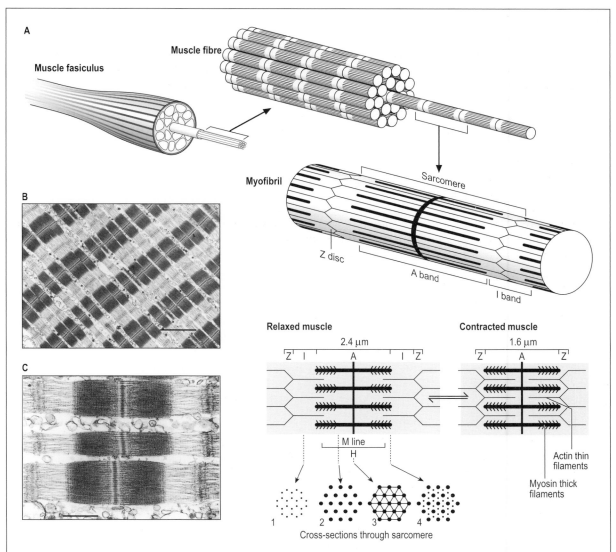

Fig. 9.11 (**A**) Organization of skeletal muscle filaments into the sliding filament model. (**B**) Electron micrograph of skeletal muscle showing regular arrangement of sarcomeres. Bar = 2 microns. (**C**) Electron micrograph showing individual sarcomeres. Bar = 500 nm. (EMs courtesy of Mrs Evaline Roberts and Dr Arthur J Rowe)

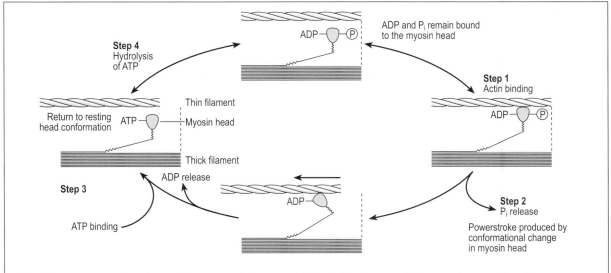

Fig. 9.12 Reaction cycle producing the powerstroke between thick and thin filaments during muscle contraction. Some conformational change contributing to the powerstroke may occur on ADP release.

113

Maintenance of phosphoryl transfer potential in muscle

Maintenance of ATP levels in muscle cells is clearly important to continued contractility. Relatively high concentrations provide a 'buffer' for phosphoryl transfer potential to maintain ATP levels required during muscular demand. Also AMP, produced by myokinase (2 ADP $\leftrightarrow$ ATP + AMP), acts as an allosteric modulator of enzymes in glycogenolysis, glycolysis, the citric acid cycle and oxidative phosphorylation, to stimulate the production of ATP.

Excitation–contraction coupling of skeletal muscle contraction

It is important for efficient contraction of skeletal muscle that the whole muscle responds in concert to a stimulus. Simple diffusion of Ca^{2+} through the tissue would be too slow to produce such a uniform response. The Ca^{2+} for contraction comes from SR Ca^{2+} stores and release is triggered by electrical activity in the sarcolemma (muscle plasma membrane). The SR of skeletal muscle is a network of membrane-delimited tubules that surrounds the myofibrils. A more regular structure of tubules is formed at the A–I band junction, which consists of two SR tubules, called terminal cisternae, separated by a deep invagination of the plasma membrane called a **transverse tubule** or **t-tubule**. The combined tubular structure is known as a **triad** (Fig. 9.13).

When an action potential passes over the surface of skeletal muscle, the t-tubular system ensures that the stimulus for contraction is transmitted rapidly deep within the fibre. L-type voltage-sensitive Ca^{2+} channels located in the t-tubule system are induced to change conformation in response to the depolarization. Rather than admit Ca^{2+} to the cell, these channels are physically coupled to ryanodine-sensitive Ca^{2+} channels in the SR and stimulate these channels to open and release Ca^{2+} from the SR store directly over the sarcomere structures that will initiate contraction (Fig. 9.14). Ca^{2+} in the cytoplasm is returned to the SR via Ca^{2+}-ATPase proteins in the SR membrane.

Malignant hyperthermia

Malignant hyperthermia is a rare, congenital condition that appears to be related to a perturbation of excitation–contraction coupling in skeletal muscle. It is induced by neuromuscular blocking drugs, e.g. suxamethonium, and volatile anaesthetics, e.g. halothane, which produce increases in $[Ca^{2+}]_i$ and skeletal muscle metabolism. Clinically, this results in intense muscle spasm and a rapid rise in body temperature and can be potentially fatal. Treatment is with dantrolene, which inhibits skeletal muscle contraction by inhibiting Ca^{2+}-induced Ca^{2+} release. The underlying cause of this autosomal dominant condition is unknown but it is noteworthy that mutations in the ryanodine-sensitive Ca^{2+} channel responsible for Ca^{2+}-induced Ca^{2+} release have been identified in patients suffering from malignant hyperthermia.

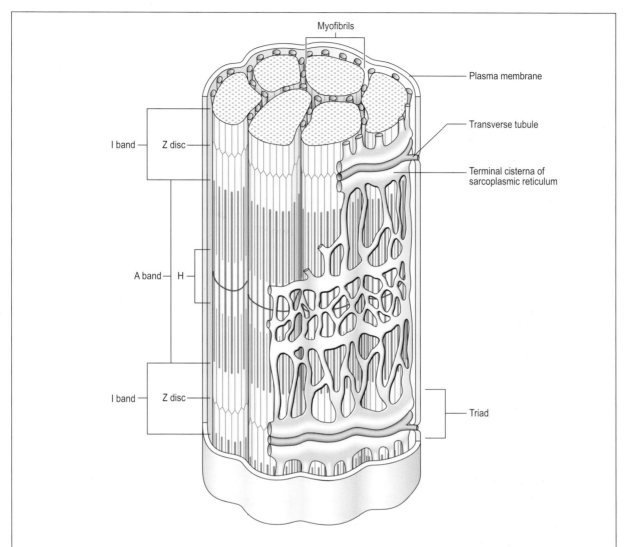

Myofibrils

Plasma membrane

Transverse tubule

Terminal cisterna of sarcoplasmic reticulum

I band — Z disc

A band — H

I band — Z disc

Triad

Fig. 9.13 Schematic diagram showing the tubular membrane network of sarcoplasmic reticulum and transverse tubules involved in coupling electrical signals to muscle contraction. Note that the sarcoplasmic reticular Ca^{2+} stores are positioned over the Ca^{2+}-sensitive microfilament regions of the sarcomere.

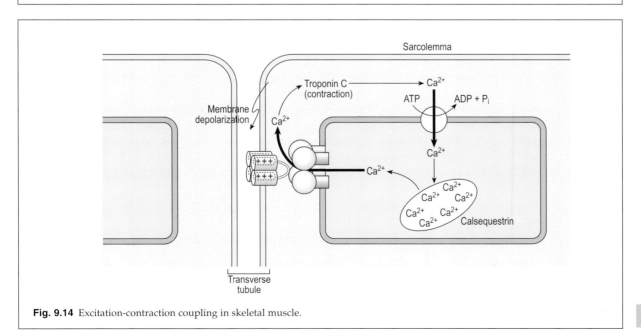

Sarcolemma

Troponin C (contraction)

Membrane depolarization

Ca^{2+}

ATP   ADP + P$_i$

Ca^{2+}

Ca^{2+}

Ca^{2+}

Ca^{2+} Ca^{2+}
Ca^{2+} Ca^{2+}
Ca^{2+} Ca^{2+}
Ca^{2+} Calsequestrin

Transverse tubule

Fig. 9.14 Excitation-contraction coupling in skeletal muscle.

Other types of muscle

Cardiac muscle

Cardiac muscle, like skeletal muscle, is composed of elongated rectangular cells with a striated appearance. The contractile machinery of the cardiac myocyte is organized into sarcomeres very similar to those seen in skeletal muscle except that cardiac-specific isoforms of the constituent proteins are involved (Fig. 9.15). Three major differences distinguish cardiac from skeletal muscle fibres:

- The nucleus in cardiac cells is positioned centrally compared with the peripheral localization under the sarcolemma in skeletal muscle fibrils.
- Cardiac muscle fibres are composed of single, mononucleated muscle cells, which are held together by specialized junctional complexes in **intercalated discs** between cells, whereas skeletal muscle consists of multinucleated fibres formed by the fusion of progenitor cells. Cardiac cells interdigitate such that intercalated disc structures form irregular junctions between transverse and longitudinal aspects of adjacent cells. Different junctional complexes contribute to different regions of the intercalated disc structures between cardiac cells. **Desmosomes** or **macula adherens** form tight structural complexes between the transverse aspect or ends of adjacent cardiac muscle cells. Also in this region are the **faciae adherens**. These structures form attachment sites for thin filaments at the sarcolemma and effectively connect the thin filaments of adjacent cells, performing a similar function to Z bands in skeletal muscle. In the longitudinal aspect of intercalated discs, **gap junctions** form. These junctions are permeable to small solutes and ions. By allowing communication between the cytoplasm of adjacent cells, these structures result in electrical coupling and, thereby, a synchronous contractile response to an initiating action potential somewhere in the tissue.
- Release of intracellular stores of Ca^{2+}, which contributes the major source of Ca^{2+} for cardiac contraction, occurs by Ca^{2+}-induced Ca^{2+} release in response to this cation entering the cell through L-type voltage-gated Ca^{2+} channels (Fig. 9.16), unlike the physical coupling of sarcolemmal L-type channels to ryanodine-sensitive Ca^{2+} channels in the SR in skeletal muscle.

Smooth muscle

Smooth muscle differs from skeletal and cardiac muscle in several ways. It is composed of elongated, tapering, single-nucleus-containing cells linked by structural junctional contacts and gap junctions (Fig. 9.17). The contractile apparatus is not arranged in sarcomeres and so the cells do not appear striated. The Ca^{2+} to initiate contraction is derived from outside the cell rather than from the SR, which is relatively poorly developed in smooth muscle. Finally, troponin is absent from smooth muscle cells and Ca^{2+} sensitivity of the contractile apparatus is conferred instead by **myosin light chain kinase (MLCK)**.

In smooth muscle the actomyosin sliding filament complexes are less organized than in striated muscle, although there is a general orientation along the axis of the cell (Fig. 9.17). The abundant thin actin filaments attach to structures called **dense bodies**, which are distributed throughout the cell. The dense bodies, like the Z band in striated muscle, are composed largely of α-actinin and the actin filaments attach by their growing ends. Dense bodies are also linked together and to the sarcolemma by a cytoskeleton of desmin and vimentin intermediate filaments. In this way contraction of the actomyosin complexes is translated to cell shortening (Fig. 9.17). Smooth muscle isoforms of actin, and particularly myosin, have similar molecular structures to other muscle forms but confer specific properties to smooth muscle. The rate of detachment of actin–myosin cross-bridges and the rate of hydrolysis of ATP by smooth muscle myosin is 10-fold lower than in striated muscle. This makes smooth muscle relatively slow to contract but allows it to maintain tension efficiently.

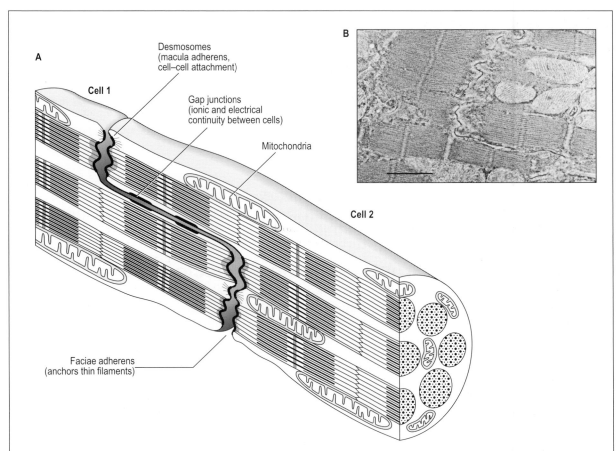

Fig. 9.15 The intercalated disc structure between cardiac muscle cells. Note: sarcomeres in adjacent cells are partially aligned. (**A**) Schematic diagram. (**B**) Electron micrograph of a thin section of cardiac muscle. Bar = 1 micron. (EM courtesy of Mrs Evaline Roberts and Dr Arthur J Rowe)

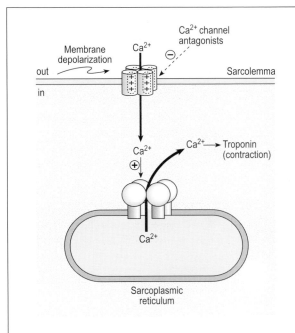

Fig. 9.16 Excitation–contraction coupling in cardiac muscle. Membrane depolarization activates voltage-gated Ca^{2+} channels in the sarcolemma. Only ~15% of the rise in $[Ca^{2+}]_i$ necessary for contraction is supplied by Ca^{2+} entry through sarcolemmal Ca^{2+} channels. The remaining Ca^{2+} is derived from the SR by Ca^{2+}-induced Ca^{2+} release.

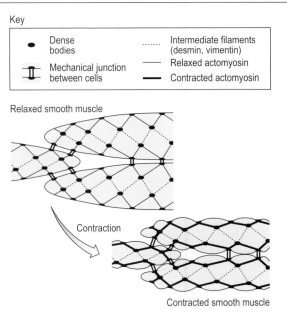

Fig. 9.17 Proposed organization of cytoskeletal elements in smooth muscle. Cell shape is maintained by a cytoskeleton of intermediate filaments linking dense bodies within the cell. On activation of myosin light chain kinase, actomyosin complexes shorten causing the cell to contract. Note: ordered sarcomere structures are not observed in smooth muscle.

117

Smooth muscle contraction depends on the phosphorylation state of myosin light chains

In smooth muscle, the interaction of myosin and actin and the ensuing contractin are dependent on the phosphorylation state of myosin light chains (Fig. 9.18). Smooth muscle myosin head groups can bind actin filaments only when the light chains are in the phosphorylated form. Like striated muscle, contraction in smooth muscle is triggered by a rise in $[Ca^{2+}]_i$. In the absence of troponin, the Ca^{2+} signal is mediated by calmodulin, which on binding Ca^{2+} activates MLCK leading to phosphorylation of myosin light chains and the binding of myosin head groups to actin filaments. When resting $[Ca^{2+}]_i$ levels are restored, the calmodulin dissociates from the MLCK rendering it inactive. Relaxation of smooth muscle also depends on a myosin light chain phosphatase to return the myosin molecule to the inactive form.

Regulation of the force of contraction in smooth muscle

Force generated by smooth muscle can be subject to negative regulation by multiple signalling pathways to produce a more relaxed state (Fig. 9.18).

Microfilamentous structures in non-muscle cells

Actomyosin structures are also found in non-muscle cells where contractile properties are required. For example, actomyosin contributes to intracellular **stress fibres**, which counter the forces imposed by the extracellular matrix. In cell culture, actomyosin is responsible for the flattening of attached cells and depolymerization results in the rounding up of cells after cell detachment. In locomotion a cell moves by extending flattened protrusions called **lamellipodia**, which form attachment sites at points of interaction with the substratum (see Figs 12.1–12.3). These structures are known to contain actin and the actin-binding proteins α-actinin and vinculin. In the retreating tail of a moving cell, depolymerization of actin filaments and formation of an actin network is thought to be important. Fungal **cytochalasins**, which bind to the growing (+) end of actin filaments and block polymerization, also block cell locomotion. Actomyosin structures are also important during telophase in the cell cycle to form the contractile ring that begins cell division (see Fig. 13.9).

Unlike striated muscle the contractile apparatus in non-muscle cells is constantly dissociating and reforming depending on the state of stimulation of the cell. In the inactive, dephosphorylated form, the myosin molecule takes up an independent globular form. On phosphorylation of the myosin light chain by MLCK, the myosin molecule extends to its rod-like form, releasing the tail domain to form bipolar thick filaments and the head domain to form cross-bridges with thin filament actin.

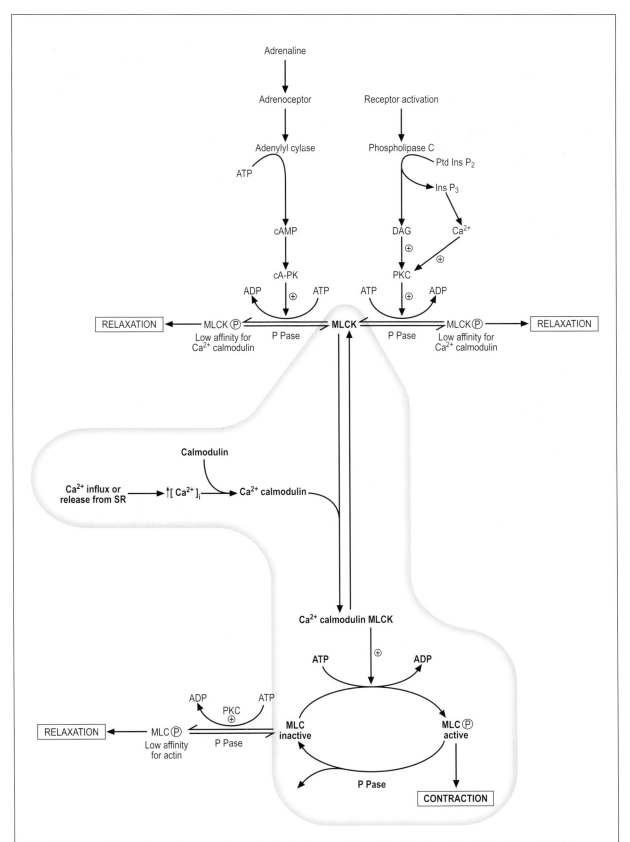

Fig. 9.18 Control of smooth muscle contraction and relaxation by regulation of the phosphorylation status of myosin light chains (MLC). The highlighted area indicates the pathway for the stimulation of smooth muscle contraction. Pathways signalling relaxation are shown in normal type. MLCK, MLC kinase; P, phosphoprotein phosphate group, cA-PK, cAMP-dependent protein kinase; PKC, protein kinase C; PPase, serine/threonine protein phosphatases; PtdlnsP$_2$, phosphatidylinositol 4,5-bisphosphate; DAG, 1,2-diacylglycerol; InsP$_3$, inositol 1,4,5-trisphosphate; cAMP, cyclic 3',5' AMP; SR, sarcoplasmic reticulum.

Microvilli

To increase the surface area of epithelial tissues the apical membrane is folded into numerous finger-like projections called **microvilli**. Microvilli are packed with bundles of actin filaments to maintain their shape (Fig. 9.19). The actin filaments are attached to the tip of each microvillus by the growing (+) end and crosslinked by the proteins fimbrin and villin. Calmodulin and a myosin-like, actin-stimulated ATPase link the actin filaments to the inner surface of the plasma membrane. Where the actin bundles protrude into the cell they interact with a meshwork structure called the **terminal web**, which is composed of actin filaments, myosin, the spectrin-like protein fodrin, α-actinin and vinculin. This structure is linked via fodrin to the cytoskeleton of intermediate filaments.

Cilia and flagella

Cilia and flagella are specialized surface appendages of cells that have a beating function (Fig. 9.20). Cilia are found grouped in ciliary fields in tissues such as pulmonary and oviduct epithelia. Synchronous beating of cilia in waves across the pulmonary epithelium permits the removal of particles from the lungs, and in the oviduct ciliary beating aids the progress of the ovum down the fallopian tube. Cilia are usually approximately 10 μm in length but they can extend up to 200 μm in some cells. In contrast, the flagellum is a long single motile element that provides a swimming mechanism. This structure is of primary importance in the swimming of spermatozoa.

Axonemal structure of cilia and flagella

Both cilia and flagella share a similar **axoneme** nine-plus-two structure based on tubulin microtubules (Fig. 9.21). These stable microtubular structures, which extend the length of the cilium or flagellum, form an array of two central tubules surrounded by nine circumferential doublet tubules. The outer doublet structures consist of a ring of 13 tubulin protofilaments (A tubule) attached to a second incomplete ring of 11 protofilaments (B tubule), which shares part of the A tubule. Each doublet is linked to the central tubules via radial spoke proteins. The doublet microtubules are also linked circumferentially by the protein **nexin**. Emanating from the A tubule of the microtubule doublets are **inner** and **outer dynein** arms. These large multisubunit proteins are composed of two or three heads attached by stalk-like structures to a basal region on the A tubule. The dynein head domains contain a myosin-like ATPase activity. When ATP binds, the dynein head groups detach from the B tubule and reattach further along the tubule. On ATP hydrolysis the dynein molecule returns to its resting conformation, which produces a sliding force between the two adjacent tubules. Longitudinal movement is restricted by the radial spokes and this produces a bend in the axoneme structure (Fig. 9.22). This mechanism must be tightly regulated so that activity occurs only in part of the structure at any one time to produce a beating motion.

Immotile cilia syndrome

Mutants in axonemal proteins can result in immotile structures (**immotile cilia syndrome**) and contribute to chronic pulmonary disorders and male infertility.

Anaesthetic depression of ciliary movement

The carpet of mucus that coats the bronchioles of the lung, trapping inhaled particles and bacteria, is normally propelled out of the lungs by ciliary beating. Anaesthetics may interfere with this by depressing ciliary motility and increasing the risk of mucous accumulation and infection in the lung.

Bacterial flagella

It is noteworthy that the structure of a bacterial flagellum is much simpler than the eukaryotic structure, consisting of a filament of a single protein that is rotated by a basal body structure at the level of the membrane. This rotation produces the characteristic spiralling motion of a moving bacterium.

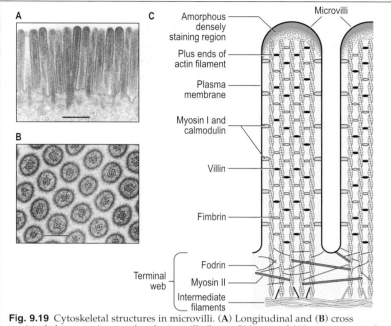

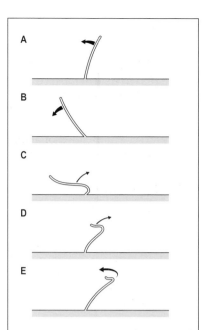

Fig. 9.19 Cytoskeletal structures in microvilli. (**A**) Longitudinal and (**B**) cross sectional electron micrographs of microvilli. Bars = 500 nm and 200 nm, respectively. (**C**) Schematic representation of arrangement of microvillus cytoskeleton. (EMs courtesy of Mrs Evaline Roberts and Dr Arthur J Rowe)

Fig. 9.20 Diagram of a ciliary beat showing the active stroke (**A** and **B**) and the recovery stroke (**C**–**E**).

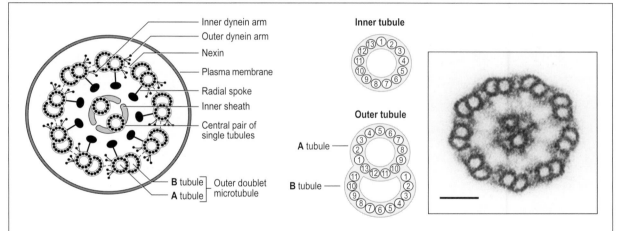

Fig. 9.21 Transverse section of a stylized cilium showing the 9 + 2 arrangement of tubules. The arrangement of individual tubule protofilaments is shown in the expanded doublet tubule. *Inset*: electron micrograph of a demembranated axoneme in transverse section. Bar = 50 nm. (EM courtesy of Mrs Evaline Roberts and Dr Arthur J Rowe)

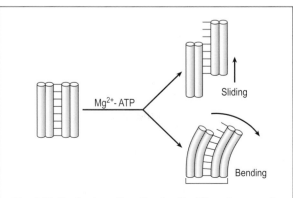

Fig. 9.22 Production of bending in cilia. When the normal longitudinal sliding movement of adjacent tubules is restricted by cross-linking structures the result of dynein 'walking' is a bend in the overall structure.

Microtubules in vesicular and organelle transport

Transport of organelles and membrane-bound vesicles in eukaryotic cells is directed along 'tracks' of single microtubules by a 'walking' mechanism. The molecular motors for this movement are myosin-like ATPases. **Kinesin** drives movement from the (–) (centrosome) end of the microtubule to the (+) end while **cytoplasmic dynein** drives movement in the opposite direction. Because microtubules are usually arranged with their centromeres near the centre of the cell, kinesin drives **anterograde** movement from the centre to the periphery, while dynein drives **retrograde** movement (Fig. 9.23). The ATP-dependent attachment of kinesin or dynein head groups with the microtubule drives the movement of the vesicle along the microtubule at up to 5 μm/s.

Kinesin is a large elongated multisubunit protein. At one end, two globular head regions provide the sites for ATP hydrolysis and cross-bridge formation to tubulin. The other flattened end interacts with proteins in the transported vesicle attaching the vesicle to the microtubular track. Unlike myosin and dynein, which release bound protein when ATP binds, the interaction of ATP with the kinesin head group promotes binding to the microtubule. Hydrolysis of the ATP molecule occurs while the microtubule is bound, causing the release of the cross-bridge and a step along the microtubule. There is considerable similarity between the structures of the kinesin and dynein head groups and the kinetics of ATP hydrolysis catalysed by the two molecules. The direction of movement of the two molecules along the microtubule may simply reflect whether the molecule walks 'forwards' or 'backwards' during the reaction cycle.

Axonal transport in neurones

Directional transport along microtubules is particularly important in the axons of neurones where cellular materials may need to be transported over relatively large distances (Fig. 9.24). Kinesin drives the fast anterograde movement of vesicles containing synaptic plasma membrane components, synaptic vesicles containing neurotransmitters and mitochondria towards the nerve terminal. Fast retrograde transport of endocytic vesicles and mitochondria is driven by dynein. In addition, axonal microtubules direct the slow unidirectional axonal transport in the anterograde direction of cytoskeletal elements such as actin, actin-binding proteins, fodrin, clathrin and cytoplasmic enzymes, and the even slower transport of cytoplasmic components such as preassembled networks of neurofilaments, microtubules and associated proteins.

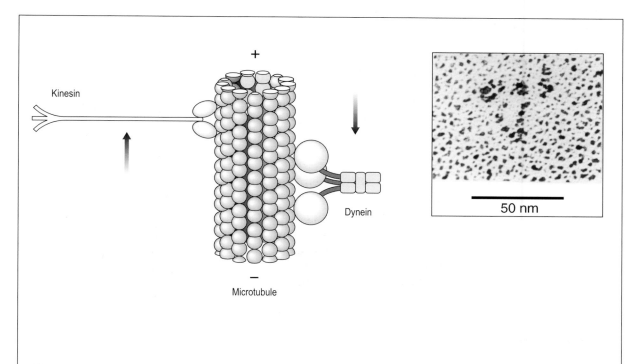

Fig. 9.23 Kinesin and dynein drive the movement of attached vesicular structures in opposite directions along microtubules. *Inset*: electron micrograph of three-headed dynein molecule. Bar = 50 nm. (EM courtesy of Dr Christine Wells)

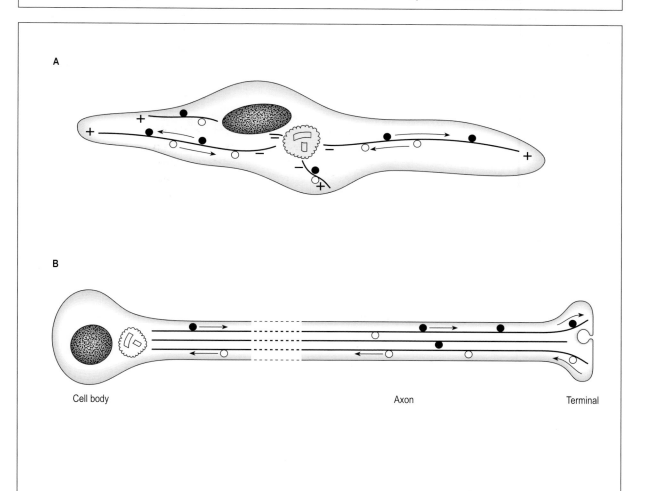

Fig. 9.24 Vesicle transport in (**A**) fibroblastic and (**B**) neuronal cells. Solid lines represent microtubules. Circles represent vesicles coated with kinesin (●) or dynein (○).

Further reading

Allen B G, Walsh M P 1994 The biochemical basis of the regulation of smooth-muscle contraction. Trends in Biochemical Sciences 19: 362–368

Bagshaw C 1993 Muscle contraction. Chapman and Hall, London

Perry S V 1996 Molecular mechanisms in striated muscle. Cambridge University Press, Cambridge

Somlyo A P, Somlyo A V 1996 Signal-transduction and regulation in smooth-muscle. Nature 372: 231–236

Vallee R B, Sheetz M P 1996 Targeting of motor proteins. Science 271: 1539–1544

Revision questions

1. Describe the basic structure of (a) microfilaments, (b) microtubules and (c) intermediate filaments. How do these structures contribute to the structure and function of cellular cytoskeletons?

2. Define the terms (a) 'myofibril', (b) 'sarcolemma', (c) 'sarcomere' and (d) 'sarcoplasm'.

3. Describe the structure of the thick and thin filaments of contractile tissues. Draw a diagram to show how these structures associate in the sarcomere. Label the following structures: 'A band', 'I band', 'H line', 'M line' and 'Z line'.

4. How is the energy of ATP hydrolysis coupled to movement in actomyosin?

5. Compare and contrast excitation–contraction coupling in skeletal, cardiac and smooth muscle.

6. What roles may actomyosin structures have in non-muscle cells?

7. How does 'treadmilling' of actin microfilaments contribute to cell locomotion? (See Chapter 12.)

8. Compare and contrast the structure and functions of cilia and flagella. What may be the physiological consequences of immotile cilia syndrome?

9. In which cytoskeletal structures is dynein found and in each case what is its function?

Answers to revision questions

1. (a) Microfilaments are helical coils of two strings of actin monomers.
   (b) Microtubules are hollow cylinders made up of 13 protofilaments of αβ tubulin dimers.
   (c) Intermediate filaments are rope-like structures composed of coiled dimers of intermediate filament proteins.
   These structures form the basic filamentous structure of cytoskeletons. They are linked by accessory proteins to other filamentous structures and to anchoring structures within the cell.

2. (a) A myofibril is the contractile element of a skeletal muscle cell.
   (b) The sarcolemma is the plasma membrane of a muscle cell.
   (c) The sarcomere is the contractile structure between two Z discs in a myofibril.
   (d) The sarcoplasm is the cytoplasm of a muscle cell.

3. Thick filaments are formed by the tail-to-tail interactions of between 300 and 400 myosin molecules to form a rigid, rod-like structure. The myosin head groups protrude from the thick filament at 60° to the next head group (see Fig. 9.9). Thin filaments are based on actin microfilaments. The exposed surface of the actin monomers is covered by tropomyosin, a long rod-like molecule that blocks the interaction of myosin in resting muscle. A second protein, troponin, is present in association with tropomyosin. Ca^{2+} binding to troponin causes the movement of tropomyosin into the groove region in the thin filament, revealing the myosin binding sites (see Fig. 9.10). Sarcomere structure is illustrated in Fig. 9.10.

4. ATP hydrolysis is required to complete the reaction cycle of myosin head group attachment to, pulling and detachment from thin filaments. Myosin head groups bind to thin filaments in the presence of bound ADP and P_i. The power stroke occurs following dissociation of P_i from the actin-bound myosin head. ADP then dissociates and the reaction cycle is blocked at this point in the absence of ATP (rigor mortis). ATP binding induces the dissociation of the myosin head group from the thin filament and its subsequent hydrolysis restores the myosin head to its actin binding conformation (see Fig. 9.12).

5. In skeletal muscle, sarcolemmal depolarization induces a conformational change in L-type Ca^{2+} channels located in the t-tubules. This change is transmitted physically to ryanodine-sensitive Ca^{2+} channels in the SR, which open to release stored Ca^{2+} to initiate contraction. In cardiac muscle, sarcolemmal depolarization stimulates the opening of L-type Ca^{2+} channels. Ca^{2+} enters the cell down its electrochemical gradient and induces Ca^{2+} release from the SR sufficient to initiate contraction. In smooth muscle, all the Ca^{2+} for contraction comes from the extracellular fluid through Ca^{2+} channels.

6. Actomyosin is found in stress fibres that counter forces imposed on cells. It is also found in the contractile ring that forms during cell division.

7. Treadmilling of the actin microfilaments results in the extension of lamellipodia and the retrograde motion of attached adhesion proteins that results in cell motion.

8. Cilia and flagella are both based on the nine-plus-two axonemal structure of tubulin microtubules. Cilia are usually relatively short (10 μm) while flagella are much longer (200 μm). Cilia are grouped in ciliary fields, while flagella are usually present as single elements. Immotile ciliary syndrome can give rise to chronic pulmonary disorders, as a result of the accumulation of mucus, and male infertility.

9. Dynein is found associated with microtubules where its function is to drive the movement of transport vesicles in a retrograde direction towards the centrosome. It is also found in the axonemal structure of cilia and flagella, associated with the outer double tubules, where it is involved in inducing a bend in the axoneme.

Adhesion molecules

A striking feature of multicellular organisms is that individual cells are differentiated, performing specific tasks, and these are arranged into discrete and highly organized functional units or tissues. The development and function of tissues is dependent on the physical interaction of one cell with another. These physical interactions are mediated by members of several families of membrane-spanning proteins, called **adhesion molecules** (Table 10.1). Adhesion molecules also play important roles in more transient interactions between cells, including those involved in cellular migration and the interactions between cells of the immune system.

Cadherins

It has been recognized for more than 30 years that cells in a suspension made from different tissues tend to sort homotypically, i.e. according to their origins. This property has since been attributed to the patterns of expression of a family of universal calcium-dependent adhesion molecules called **cadherins** (Fig. 10.1A) that mediate homotypic cell–cell adhesion. The preference of a cell for other cells from the same tissue appears to depend not only on the types(s) of cadherin expressed but also on their relative abundance. There are many different subgroups of cadherin, each with distinct functions and patterns of expression, all encoded by different genes. Structurally, all cadherins have five extracellular domains, four of which are homologous and are thought to bind Ca^{2+}. Removal of Ca^{2+} causes a conformational change that makes the molecule protease-sensitive. X-ray crystallographic data suggest that cadherins form dimers, with their binding domains facing away from each other allowing each pair to interact with those on neighbouring cells (Fig. 10.1B). The intracellular domain (there may be different forms for each family member, produced by alternative splicing) is responsible for binding to complexes of cytoplasmic plaque proteins, which link cadherins to the actin cytoskeleton (**adherens junctions**) or intermediate filaments (**desmosomes**), and for signal transduction. The ability of cadherins to become linked to actin and intermediate filaments allows neighbouring cells to form strong structures, such as epithelial sheets, by joining their cytoskeletons together to form transcellular networks.

Integrins

Cells not only interact physically with each other but also with the **extracellular matrix** (ECM). The ECM is a mass of proteins and polysaccharides found in the gaps between cells, which provides elasticity and resistance to tensile and compressing forces (see Chapter 11). In some cases ECM proteins are organized into specialized structures called basement membranes, which provide a physical barrier separating epithelial and endothelial cells from the underlying mesenchymal tissues. A second family of adhesion molecules, the **integrins** are responsible for many of the interactions between cells and the ECM. Integrins are membrane-anchored heterodimeric glycoproteins. Each one consists of non-covalently associated α and β subunits (Fig. 10.2), both of which play a part in ligand binding. So far 16 different α and nine different β subunits have been identified, giving the potential for a large number of distinct dimers, although only a limited number of combinations have been identified in vivo. Both integrin subunits have cytoplasmic domains that are important for signal transduction and the formation of anchoring junctions. In addition to mediating cell–matrix interactions in adherens junctions and **hemi-desmosomes**, a subgroup of integrins (those containing β_2) can also form cell–cell interactions by acting as **counter-receptors** (ligands) for a third class of adhesion molecules, which are members of the **immunoglobulin superfamily**. The diversity of adhesive contacts formed by integrins means that they do not simply hold tissues together, but also contribute to a wide range of physiological processes including cell migration, wound healing, adhesion of leucocytes to activated endothelium, phagocytosis, platelet aggregation and T cell functions. These diverse functions are illustrated by several inherited disorders that result from defects in integrin expression (Table 10.2).

Family	Examples	Ca^{2+}-dependence	Major ligands	Cell Types	Main functions
Cadherin	E	+	Self	Epithelial	Cell–cell junctions
	N	+	Self	Nerve, muscle	Cell–cell junctions
	P	+	Self	Placental, epidermal	Cell–cell junctions
Integrin	β_1	+	ECM	All cells	Cell–matrix junctions
	β_2	+	Ig superfamily	Leucocytes	Inflammation, T cell interactions and lymphocyte homing
	β_3	+	ECM	Platelets and others	Blood clotting
Selectin	P	+	sLe^x, sLe^a	Platelets, endothelial	Inflammation
	E	+	sLe^x, sLe^a	Endothelial	Inflammation
	L	+	sLe^x, sLe^a	Leucocytes	Inflammation and lymphocyte homing
Immunoglobulin	ICAM	−	β_2 integrin	Lymphocytes, endothelial	Inflammation, T cell interactions and lymphocyte homing
	VCAM	−			
	NCAM	−	Self	Nerves	Neural development

Table 10.1 Adhesion molecules: the characteristics of the four main families of adhesion molecule. sLe^x, sialyl Lewis^x; sLe^a, sialyl Lewis^a

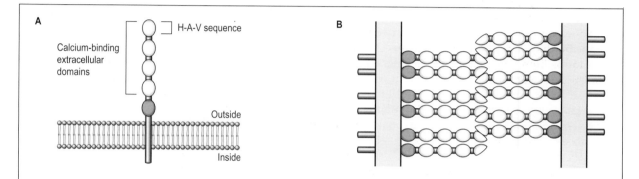

Fig. 10.1 (**A**) Cadherin structure: a schematic diagram of a cadherin homodimer, showing five extracellular domains. Four of the extracellular domains (EC1–4) are homologous and bind calcium. Dimers are thought to form with their binding faces (which contain a conserved histidine-alanine-valine [H-A-V] motif) facing away from each other. (**B**) Model of cadherin-mediated intercellular adhesion: X-ray diffraction studies suggest that cadherin dimers on adjacent cells are bound together by the interaction of their EC1 domains, thus forming zip-like structures.

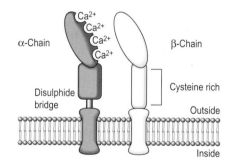

Fig. 10.2 Integrin structure: A schematic diagram of an integrin $\alpha\beta$ heterodimer. The alpha subunit, carries four binding sites for divalent cations. In certain cases (e.g. α_3, α_5, α_6, α_7) alpha subunits are cleaved to form two disulphide-linked peptides. Other alpha subunits (e.g. α_1, α_2, α_L, α_M) have an insertion of 200 amino acids (I domain) near the N-terminal.

Adhesion molecule	Disease	Defect	Consequence	Symptoms
Integrin β_2	Lymphocyte adhesion deficiency 1	Splicing defect in integrin β_2 prevents surface expression.	Deficiency in leucocyte infiltration to sites of inflammation	Recurrent infection
Integrin β_3	Glanzman's thromblasthenia	Integrin β_3 is absent – platelets lack fibrinogen receptor	Platelets do not aggregate in response to agonist	Severe bleeding
Integrin $\alpha_6\beta_4$	Junctional epidermolysis bullosa	Deficiency in expression of integrin $\alpha_6\beta_4$	Reduction in binding of squamous epithelia to basement membranes	Blistering of skin

Table 10.2 Inherited disorders caused by integrin deficiency

> **Integrins and thrombosis**
>
> The integrin gpIIb/IIIa ($\alpha_{IIb}\beta_3$) expressed on the surface of platelets acts as a receptor for fibrinogen and von Willebrand factor and mediates the aggregation of platelets in response to stimulation by agonist. An anti-gpIIb/IIIa antibody has been shown to be a powerful anti-thrombotic and is useful in the prevention of ischaemic complications following percutaneous transluminal coronary angioplasty.

Immunoglobulin superfamily

The immunoglobulin (Ig) superfamily is a large, diverse family (> 70 members) of proteins, with a complex array of structures, which includes several Ca^{2+}-independent adhesion molecules (Fig. 10.3). All contain a basic motif of 70–110 amino acids, forming two parallel sheets usually stabilized by disulphide bridges (the immunoglobulin fold). In addition to acting as counter-receptors for β2 integrins, Ig superfamily molecules (Fig. 10.3) on one cell may bind to identical molecules on another cell (**homotypic binding**), and to other members of the family. Family members (known as **cellular adhesion molecules** or CAMs) play important roles in T cell interactions (ICAM-1, inter-CAM) and in the binding of leucocytes to activated (ICAM-1; VCAM-1, vascular CAM) and resting (ICAM-2) endothelium. One of the most widely expressed Ig superfamily molecules is NCAM (neural CAM), which appears to play an important role in the developing nervous system. The degree of post-translational modification of NCAM molecules, by the addition of sialic acid residues, may be an important mechanism for determining whether NCAM promotes adhesion (as it does in linking nerve cell processes to form bundles (axonal fasciculation)) or possibly inhibits it (which favours nerve process outgrowth).

Organization of cells into tissues

Tight junctions

Tight (or occluding) junctions can be impermeable even to small molecules (although this varies according to the tissue). This property allows epithelial cells that are linked by tight junctions to form sheets, and to act as permeability barriers. However, tight junctions are not simply fixed structures: the degree of permeability is under physiological control, responding to intracellular signals. The best-studied tight junctions are those joining the epithelial cells that form the lining of the gut (Fig. 10.4). Here solutes leaving the digestive system must traverse the epithelial cells in order to reach the bloodstream, allowing these cells to control which molecules are absorbed. Tight junctions also permit the apical and basolateral domains of the plasma membrane, which interface with different physiological compartments, to be separated. This allows specialization of the domains, and prevents their different transporter proteins from becoming mixed. A possible model of tight junction structure is shown in Fig. 10.5.

Anchoring junctions

Anchoring junctions are responsible for maintaining the integrity of tissues. They achieve this by linking the cytoskeletons of adjoining cells to each other, or to the ECM. Adherens junctions contain links to actin and desmosomes and hemi-desmosomes to intermediate filaments. All anchoring junctions share a similar basic structure with the link between membrane-spanning adhesion molecules (cadherin or integrin) and the cytoskeleton being provided by groups of cytoplasmic plaque proteins (Fig. 10.6). The prevalence of anchoring junctions depends on the degree to which a tissue is subjected to mechanical stress. For example, skin epithelium, which is under constant strain, has large numbers of such structures.

Adherens junctions

Cell–cell. In non-epithelial tissues these junctions may be punctate or appear streak-like, but in epithelial tissues they form continuous belts around the entire circumference of each cell. Cells are linked by cadherins. The cytoplasmic domains of the cadherin molecules are bound to three

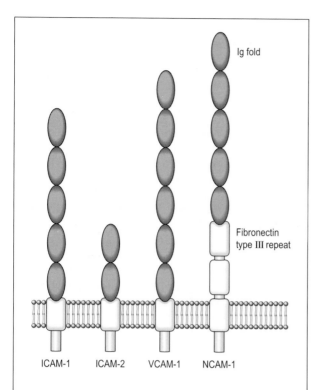

Fig. 10.3 Examples of immunoglobulin (Ig) superfamily adhesion molecules: intercellular adhesion molecule 1 (ICAM-1), intercellular adhesion molecule 2 (ICAM-2), vascular cell adhesion molecule 1 (VCAM-1) and neural cell adhesion molecule-1 (NCAM).

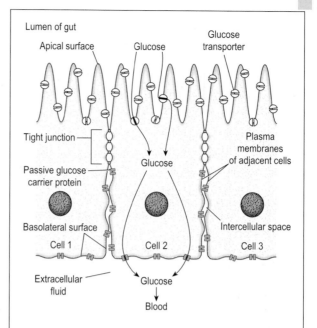

Fig. 10.4 Schematic diagram of gut epithelium showing how tight junctions act as permeability barriers, allowing compartmentalization of tissues, and also segregation of the apical and basolateral domains of the plasma membrane with their different membrane proteins (in this case the apical glucose transporter, which acts against the concentration gradient to take up glucose from the gut, and the basolateral glucose carrier which allows it to enter the bloodstream by facilitated diffusion) thus permitting the vectorial uptake of solutes into the blood.

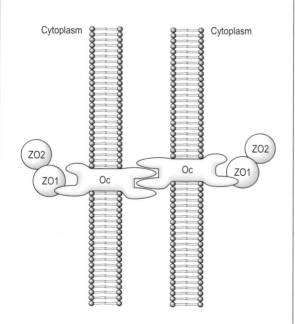

Fig. 10.5 A possible model of tight junction structure. Tight junctions are formed by the integral membrane protein occludin (Oc). Each junction is made up of many occludin molecules arranged in rows like stitching in a seam. Various additional proteins are associated with tight junctions; ZO1, which is necessary for the incorporation of occludin into tight junctions, binds to its carboxy terminus. A second, homologous, accessory protein, ZO2, is associated with ZO1.

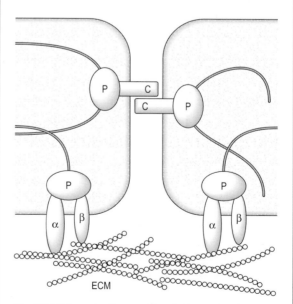

Fig. 10.6 Schematic diagram of anchoring junctions. Cell–cell junctions are made by cadherins (C) and cell–matrix junctions mostly by integrins ($\alpha\beta$). These are linked by complexes of cytoplasmic plaque proteins (P) either to the actin cytoskeleton (adherens junctions) or to intermediate filaments (desmosomes and hemi-desmosomes). Although the different types of anchoring junction have similar structures, the distance between adhering cells is greater at desmosomes (25 nm) than at adherens junctions (20 nm). ECM, extracellular matrix.

cytoplasmic plaque proteins (β-catenin, plakoglobin and p120). This complex is linked by α-catenin to the actin filament bundles, which lie parallel to the plasma membrane. The association of cadherins with the cytoskeleton through adherens junctions not only helps to stabilize structures such as epithelial sheets but is also thought to allow them to fold, taking on different morphological forms, in response to contraction of the cytoskeleton.

Cell–matrix. In certain cell types, specialized junctions form in specific regions of the plasma membrane where actin bundles terminate. These junctions are called **focal adhesions** or **focal contacts**. Focal adhesion assembly involves binding of integrins to the ECM, followed by clustering of integrins and binding of cytoplasmic plaque proteins (including talin, vinculin and α-actinin), which provide a link to the cytoskeleton. Locally generated intracellular signals (including phosphorylation by several kinases, e.g. focal adhesion kinase and phosphatidylinositol 3-kinase) are also thought to play an important role in controlling the integrity of focal adhesions. Exerting control over the making and breaking of ECM contacts is obviously vital in providing traction for migrating cells. Other adhesion molecules may also mediate interactions between cells and the ECM. For example, integral membrane **proteoglycans**, the **syndecans**, may be found in focal adhesions. In skeletal muscle the major link between the actin cytoskeleton and the ECM involves **dystroglycan**, a glycoprotein, which is an adhesion receptor for **laminin**. Dystroglycan forms part of a membrane complex of proteins that are connected to actin by a cytoplasmic plaque protein, **dystrophin**. Mutations that affect the stability of dystrophin are responsible for **Duchenne muscular dystrophy**, a severe muscle-wasting disorder (Fig. 10.7).

Desmosomes and hemi-desmosomes

Desmosomes (Fig. 10.8) are formed from cadherin-linked complexes of cytoplasmic plaque proteins which act as anchoring sites for intermediate filaments. This allows the intermediate filaments to form a strong transcellular network giving the tissue resistance to shear stress. Recent evidence suggests that desmosomes contribute more than just mechanical strength, with certain components having roles in signal transduction. Structurally, desmosomes resemble rivets with protein plaques (including plakoglobin and desmoplakin) in each cell, linked by membrane-spanning cadherins (called desmogleins and desmocollins).

Hemi-desmosomes link cells to the ECM by anchoring the network of intermediate filaments, providing extra strength. As their name implies they are morphologically similar to desmosomes but the composition of hemi-desmosome plaques is different and the link to the matrix is provided by integrins (principally $\alpha_6\beta_4$, which binds to laminin in the basement membrane).

Distribution of cell junctions

Each of the six types of cell junction (Fig. 10.9) has a different function and their relative abundance and distribution reflects the differing needs of the cell.

Regulation of adhesion

Whilst the integrity of a mature tissue depends on its constituent cells being locked into place by adhesive interactions, cell migration is essential not just in development but also in normal growth, wound healing, tissue remodelling and in the immune system. Migration is also heavily dependent on adhesive interactions to provide traction for the cell, but here the emphasis is on cell–matrix rather than cell–cell interactions. One obvious way in which adhesion can be regulated is by controlling the surface expression of adhesion molecules either by inducing gene expression or by mobilizing intracellular stores of preformed molecules. Many morphological processes in embryo development appear to be controlled at least in part by the modulation of cadherin gene expression. For example, neural crest cells transiently stop expression of N-cadherin prior to separating from the neural tube but then start re-expressing it before reassociating together once they have left the tube. However, other mechanisms are likely to play an important role. For example, it has been shown recently that cultured human breast epithelial cells, transformed with an activated form of the oncogene *ras*, switch from a non-invasive to a highly invasive form. This switch is characterized by a change in the predominant form of adhesive contact from adherens junctions (cell–cell) to focal contacts (cell–matrix).

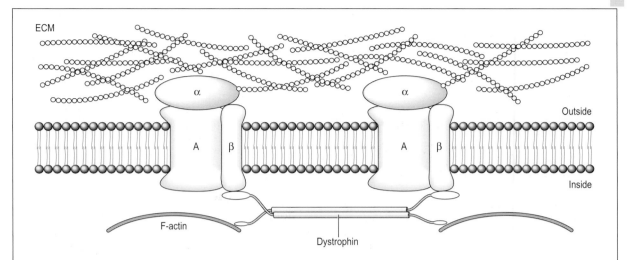

Fig. 10.7 Muscular dystrophy. Dystrophin (possibly in the form of a dimer) links F-actin (the precise location of the actin-binding site on dystrophin has yet to be established unequivocally) to the extracellular matrix protein laminin via a glycoprotein complex including α-dystroglycan (α), β-dystroglycan (β) and several other membrane proteins (A). Patients with Duchenne muscular dystrophy lack functional dystrophin. Other muscular dystrophies may arise from deficiences in other components of the link (e.g. see Chapter 11). A possible explanation of the pathology is that the loss of this stabilizing interaction makes the muscle fibres vulnerable to the mechanical stress caused by muscle contraction. ECM, extracellular matrix.

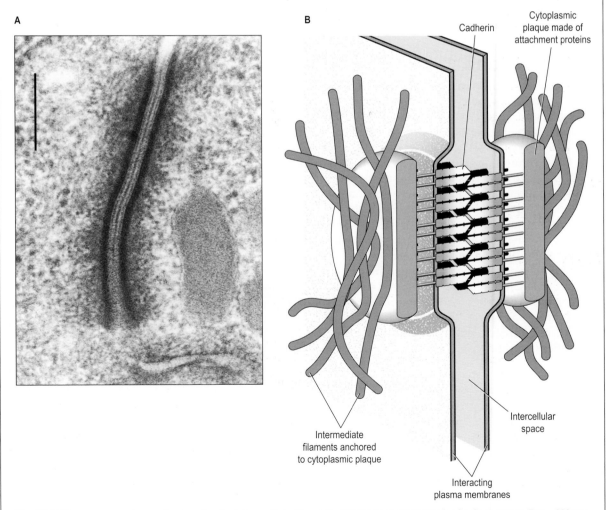

Fig. 10.8 Desmosomes act as anchoring sites for intermediate filaments. (**A**) Electron micrograph of a desmosome. Bar = 200 nm. (**B**) Schematic diagram of a desmosome. (EM courtesy of Mrs Evaline Roberts and Dr Arthur J Rowe)

Adhesion molecules as signal transducers

As can be seen with the regulation of focal adhesions, binding of adhesion molecules to their ligands is not just an isolated event. For example, the avidity with which leucocyte integrins bind to activated vascular endothelium can be modulated by activation of intracellular signalling pathways by chemoattractants or cytokines. The integrin molecules respond to an intracellular event by adopting a new, more adhesive conformation (Fig. 10.10). This process, where a cell's interactions with its extracellular environment respond to an intracellular event, is referred to as inside-out signalling. In addition to allowing the cell to respond to extracellular signals by modulating adhesiveness, integrins also contribute to the intracellular response to extracellular events. Not only does binding of ligand appear to lead to integrin clustering and focal adhesion assembly, but there is also strong evidence that adhesion molecules have a role in signal transduction in many important cellular processes, in addition to those regulating adhesion and migration. For example, it has been shown in culture that the mitogenic response of cells, such as fibroblasts, to growth factors is dependent on adhesion to the ECM (Fig. 10.11).

Adhesion molecules also participate in the regulation of apoptosis and the expression of specific genes (e.g. the cytoplasmic plaque proteins β-catenin and plakoglobin can translocate to the nucleus and interact with certain transcription factors). It has been shown that certain genes are dependent on the presence of the ECM for their transcription. For example, expression of the albumin gene in hepatocytes is regulated by attachment to the ECM. The simplest model is that binding to the ECM regulates either the expression or the activity of specific transcription factors, which in turn activate transcription of the regulated gene by binding to an ECM-response element. As with the mitogenic response of cells to growth factors, the tissue-specific and developmental regulation of certain genes (for example, the milk protein β-casein gene in mammary epithelial cells) appears to require both the presence, and the integration, of several distinct signals, and may in addition require the cell to adopt a particular morphological organization.

Gap junctions

In common with synapses, **gap junctions** are a type of **communicating junction**. Gap junctions are pores that link the cytoplasm of adjacent cells together. These pores are large enough to allow molecules up to 1000 Da to pass freely from cell to cell. This is sufficient to allow the passage of inorganic ions (Na^+, K^+, Ca^{2+}) and small organic molecules such as amino acids or second messengers such as cyclic AMP, cyclic GMP or $InsP_3$, but not macromolecules such as proteins or nucleic acids. These connections between cells mean that they can be coupled both chemically (or metabolically) and electrically. This helps a tissue to respond as an integrated unit rather than as individual cells and is important in synchronizing the contraction of myocytes to produce a beat in cardiac muscle. Gap junctions play an important role in embryogenesis, and gap junction dysfunction may also be involved in cancer.

Gap junctions are formed where structures called **connexons** from adjacent cells meet to form a pore (Fig. 10.12). Connexons are made up of six identical protein subunits (**connexins**), which each have four membrane-spanning domains. There are several different forms of connexin encoded by different genes. This provides for a diversity of gap junctions each with a different tissue distribution and each with slightly different properties. It is not clear whether different connexins can combine to produce a functional gap junction. In common with ion channels, connexons are gated, i.e. their opening is regulated. In the case of gap junctions it is thought that this regulation may be by cytosolic pH or Ca^{2+} concentration. Reductions in intracellular pH or increases in Ca^{2+} cause the pores to close.

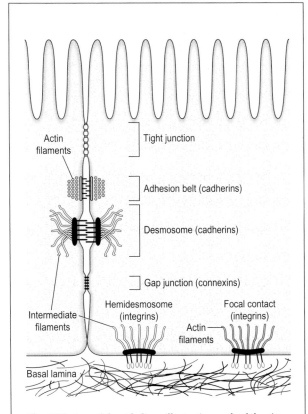

Fig. 10.9 A model epithelium illustrating each of the six distinct types of cell–cell and cell–matrix junctions.

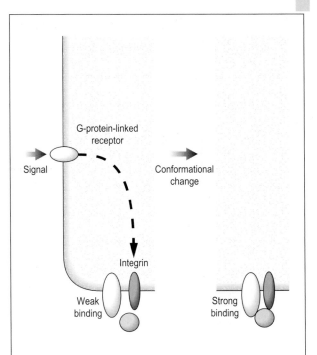

Fig. 10.10 Modulation of integrin affinity. Integrin molecules respond to an intracellular signal (in this case generated in response to binding of ligand to a G-protein-linked receptor) by adopting a new more adhesive conformation. This is thought to involve a stimulus to their cytoplasmic domains, possibly phosphorylation, binding of calcium or another protein.

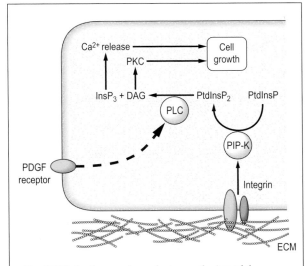

Fig. 10.11 Anchorage-dependent growth. A model explaining how the mitogenic response of fibroblasts to platelet-derived growth factor (PDGF) is modulated by attachment to the extracellular matrix (ECM). Binding of PDGF to its receptor leads to the activation of phospholipase C (PLC). In adherent cells (bound to fibronectin), integrin clustering causes activation of phosphatidylinositol phosphate 5-kinase (PIP-K) and production of phosphatidylinositol 4,5 bisphosphate (PdtlnsP$_2$) from phosphatidylinositol 4-phosphate (PdtlnsP). PdtlnsP$_2$ is metabolized by PLC to form diacylglycerol (DAG), which activates protein kinase C (PKC), and inositol trisphosphate (InsP$_3$) which triggers calcium release. Non-adherent cells have low levels of PdtlnsP$_2$ and are, therefore, insensitive to growth factor-induced activation of PLC.

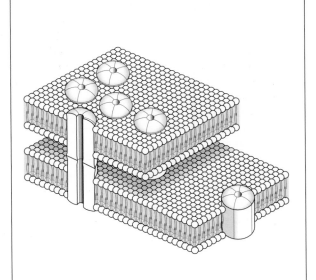

Fig. 10.12 Gap junctions are pores formed where connexons (complexes of six membrane-spanning proteins called connexins) from adjacent cells meet. Under the electron microscope gap junctions differ from tight junctions in that a small uniform gap (2 nm) is seen between the plasma membranes of the connected cells. Consequently, gap junctions do not restrict the movement of molecules in the intercellular space (in between cells).

Adhesion molecules in the immune system

In addition to the many chemical interactions between cells of the immune system, physical interactions play several vital roles. Cell–cell and cell–matrix contacts are important for the process of immune surveillance, whereby immune cells patrol the tissues looking for foreign antigens or damage. Once such stimuli are encountered, there is a need to recruit large numbers of cells to the site as part of the inflammatory response. Again, cell adhesion is essential. The interactions between helper T cells and both antigen-presenting and B cells also involve adhesion molecules, including LFA-1 (T cells) and ICAM-1, ICAM-2 and ICAM-3 (B cells and antigen-presenting cells).

Immune surveillance of the tissues

Lymphocytes periodically leave the circulation and enter the tissues. This process is non-random with cells being able to migrate into selected tissues and to locate specific microenvironments within them (a process referred to as **ecotaxis**). The function of the immune system is to differentiate between self and non-self, but immune cells are also able to tell one part of self from another. This allows them to locate themselves precisely within a tissue, returning or 'homing' to specific peripheral lymphoid organs. Circulating lymphocytes are guided to specific parts of the body by their recognition of **addressins** or homing receptors expressed by specialized blood vessels called high endothelial venules, through which they leave the circulation. Some of these addressin molecules have been identified as sialylated carbohydrates of the **sialyl Lewis^x** type, which act as ligands for an adhesion molecule called **L-selectin** carried by the lymphocyte. L-selectin, which also binds sulphated carbohydrates, is one of three members of a family of membrane-anchored proteins that share a high degree of homology (Fig. 10.13). The additional members, E-selectin (expressed by activated vascular endothelium) and P-selectin (expressed by platelets and activated vascular endothelium) play an important role in inflammation.

Inflammation

The mounting of a successful immune response is dependent on the recruitment of large numbers of leucocytes (particularly neutrophils) to the site of inflammation. These cells must attach themselves to vascular endothelial cells and then migrate into the tissues. Neutrophils leave the circulation in a multistep process, which involves three families of adhesion molecule (Fig. 10.14).

Adhesion molecules and inflammatory disease

Tissue eosinophilia is a feature of allergic inflammatory diseases, such as asthma and nasal polyposis. Selective blocking of eosinophil interactions with activated endothelium by antagonists such as anti-P-selectin or anti-integrin $\alpha_4\beta_7$ monoclonal antibodies may form the basis for future therapeutic options.

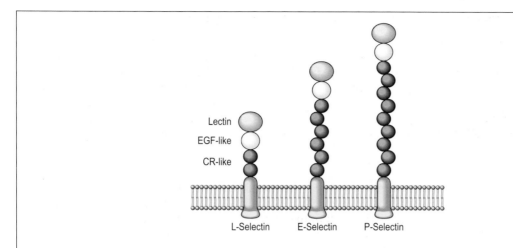

Fig. 10.13 Selectins have three types of extracellular domain: a carbohydrate-binding lectin domain, a domain homologous to a repeat found in epidermal growth factor (EGF) (which also contributes to binding), and a variable number of repeats of a sequence found in complement regulatory (CR) proteins. Selectins bind to sialylated carbohydrates of the sialyl Lewis^x type. Sialyl Lewis^x is a tetrasaccharide containing sialic acid, galactose, fucose and N-acetyl glucosamine.

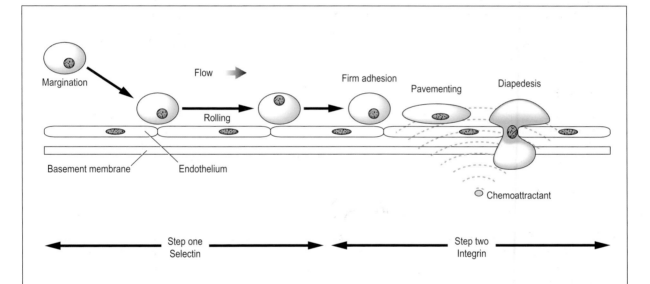

Fig. 10.14 Leucocytes leaving a blood vessel in response to an inflammatory stimulus. There are two distinct phases of adhesion, each mediated by different families of adhesion molecule. The first step involves selectin-mediated rolling of neutrophils along activated endothelium. The second step involves arrest and firm adhesion mediated by the interaction of neutrophil integrins ($\alpha_L\beta_2/\alpha_M\beta_2$. $\alpha_4\beta_1$) with members of the immunoglobulin superfamily (ICAM-1, VCAM-1) expressed on endothelial cells. Firmly adhered cells change shape, flattening themselves against the side of the blood vessel, and then migrate through the endothelium into the tissues (diapedesis). Migration through the endothelial layer involves the interaction of ICAM-1 with $\alpha_L\beta_2$.

Further reading

Pigott R, Power C 1993 The adhesion molecule factsbook. Academic Press, London

Gumbiner B M 1996 Cell adhesion: the molecular basis of tissue architecture and morphogenesis. Cell 84: 345–357

Kumar N M, Gilula N B 1996 The gap junction communication channel. Cell 84: 381–388

Revision questions

1. How do the adhesive contacts of migrating and non-motile cells differ?

2. What is anchorage-dependent growth?

3. Describe the different ways in which cell adhesiveness might be regulated.

4. The cytoplasmic domains of integrins have several important functions. What are they?

5. Gap junctions and tight junctions may both allow the passage of certain molecules, but how do they differ fundamentally?

Answers to revision questions

1. In non-motile cells, adherens junctions (cell–cell) predominate, whereas motile cells form more focal contacts (cell–matrix).

2. The ability of certain cells to respond positively to growth factors is dependent on the integration of more than one signal. For example, growth may only occur when the cell is appropriately attached to the ECM.

3. Adhesion could be regulated by controlling the surface expression of adhesion molecules by inducing or repressing gene expression, by mobilizing intracellular stores of preformed molecules, by increasing turnover, or by altering adhesion molecule conformation and therefore affinity, e.g. by phosphorylation.

4. The cytoplasmic domains allow the integrins to be linked to the cytoskeleton by the formation of anchoring junctions, and play an important role in signal transduction allowing the cell to sense its environment and to respond to stumuli by modulating its adhesiveness.

5. Gap junctions permit movement of intracellular solutes from one cell another, whereas tight junctions regulate the movement of solutes from one compartment to another through intercellular spaces.

The extracellular matrix

Cells make up only a proportion of tissues. Much of the human body is comprised of connective tissues, which contain few cells. Connective tissues are chiefly made from extracellular matrix (ECM), a mass of specialized proteins and polysaccharides mainly secreted by fibroblasts. Certain tissues such as skin or bone, which have major structural roles, contain a high proportion of connective tissue, whereas neural tissue, which has no structural role, contains very little. As illustrated by anchorage-dependent growth (Chapter 10), the ECM does not simply provide a protective framework but also has a profound influence on the behaviour of individual cells.

Collagen

Members of the **collagen** family of fibrous proteins (Table 11.1) are the most abundant proteins in mammals, (accounting for 25% of total protein) and are major components of skin and bone. There are many collagens and other proteins with collagen-like domains characterized by large numbers of repeats of the sequence Gly-X-Y (where X is usually proline and Y often hydroxyproline or hydroxylysine). These domains form a tight coil (left-handed helix) with glycine on the inside and the larger residues on the outside. The basic unit of collagen is a triple helix (right-handed) of three of these polypeptides (α-chain) wound together. Many different α-chains have been identified, each encoded by a separate gene. Combinations of distinct α-chains aggregate together to form the different fibrillar and non-fibrillar types of collagen.

Collagen biosynthesis

Collagens are extensively post-translationally modified. Translation occurs on ribosomes bound to the ER (see Chapter 5). Fibrillar and many non-fibrillar collagens are synthesized as procollagens with non-helix-forming domains at their N- and C-terminal ends. These propeptides are released into the lumen of the ER where the signal sequences are cleaved. The resulting pro α-chains are then heavily modified, by hydroxylation of selected proline and lysine residues and also by glycosylation. The C-termini of three molecules then associate and link by the formation of disulphide bonds, and the helical domains autoassemble into the characteristic triple helical α-chain. To avoid polymerization occurring within the cell, the non-helical regions of fibrillar procollagens are retained until after the molecule has been secreted. This ensures that damaging fibrils do not form within the cell. Whilst the procollagen molecules are still associated with the cell, usually in a membrane fold, the propeptides are removed by secreted proteinases and the molecules are crosslinked together to form fibrils (Fig. 11.1). Collagen fibrils, which have a regular structure of overlapping collagen molecules, can aggregate together to form collagen fibres. Collagen fibres are laid down in an ordered fashion by fibroblasts, which exert tension on the growing fibre to ensure it lies in the appropriate orientation (relative to the anticipated shearing forces). In bone, sheets of type I (fibrous) collagen are laid down with the fibres of succeeding layers at right angles to the previous one. This arrangement ensures considerable strength.

Elastin

Whilst collagen provides tissues with tensile strength, **elastin** is responsible for giving them elasticity. Like collagen, elastin contains large numbers of glycine and proline residues but its structure is much less regular. Elastic fibres are made up of crosslinked elastin monomers and microfibrillar proteins such as fibrillin. In the absence of stress, the elastin molecules are thought to have a globular structure but under tension they stretch, becoming more linear (Fig. 11.2).

Collagen	Type	Structure	Expression
Fibril forming	I, II, III, V, XI	Fibres	Connective tissues, cartilage
Network forming	IV, VIII, X	Sheets	Basement membranes, endothelium
Fibril associated	IX, XII, XIV, XVI, XIX	Link to fibrils	Connective tissues, cartilage
Anchoring fibril forming	VII	Dimers anchoring basement membranes to ECM	Basement membranes

Table 11.1 Types of collagen and the structures they form. ECM, extracellular matrix

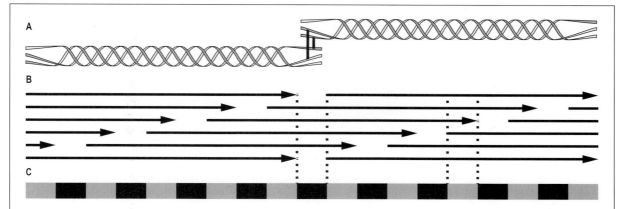

Fig. 11.1 (**A**) Collagen fibrils. Individual triple helices are stabilized by internal covalent bonds and α-chains are linked together by interchain bonds between the non-helical ends of neighbouring chains. (**B**) A collagen fibril made up of overlapping covalently linked collagen α-chains. (**C**) Under the electron microscope, collagen fibrils show a characteristic striped appearance. This is because the gaps between α-chains, which absorb the negative stain used in this technique, are aligned in these structures.

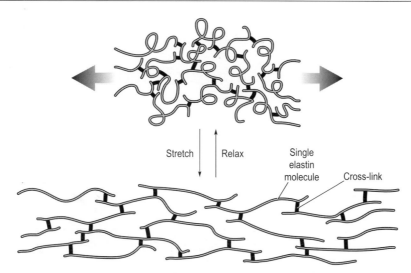

Fig. 11.2 A network of covalently linked elastin molecules provides elasticity. When stretched, the molecules elongate, absorbing energy. When allowed to relax, they revert to a more globular structure.

Fibronectin

Fibronectin (Fig. 11.3) is a large disulphide-linked dimeric glycoprotein which plays key roles in cell adhesion and migration in development, malignancy, blood clotting, host defence and in the maintenance of tissue integrity. There are two forms of fibronectin: plasma fibronectin (produced by hepatocytes and secreted into the bloodstream) and cellular fibronectin (produced mainly by fibroblasts) which forms part of the ECM. Fibronectin has binding sites for collagen, integrins (two sites), heparin and fibrin. There are, in fact, several different forms arising from alternative splicing (see Chapter 2) in three regions of the fibronectin transcript. The precise differences in function between isoforms are unclear at present, but the balance of expression does vary from one cell type to another, and according to circumstance. For example, certain exons are included in fibronectin produced during embryogenesis or during repair of damaged tissue, but excluded from fibronectin found in normal adult tissue.

Laminin

Laminin is the first ECM protein to be detected during embryogenesis and plays a vital role in neuronal outgrowth and nerve regeneration. It is a large glycoprotein in the shape of an asymmetric cross (Fig. 11.4) and is composed of three different disulphide-linked chains (α, β and γ). Laminin monomers self-associate (via the N-terminal globular domains of the three chains) to form mesh-like networks, which contribute to the structure of basal laminae (see below). There are variants of each chain, giving rise to several unique laminin isoforms, with differing distribution and function. Like fibronectin, laminin is a multidomain protein and is able to bind several other ECM components including type IV collagen, heparin, and nidogen (also known as enactin). The α chain of laminin can bind to laminin cell surface receptor proteins including certain integrins (e.g. $\alpha_6\beta_1$ and $\alpha_1\beta_2$) and α-dystroglycan which binds the α_2 chain.

Alzheimer's disease

Unusually high levels of laminin have been reported in the brains of patients suffering from Alzheimer's disease. The increased laminin expression is associated with the senile plaques and co-localizes with β-amyloid protein. Precisely how abnormal laminin expression might contribute to the pathology of this disease is unclear at present.

Proteoglycans and glycosaminoglycans

Glycosaminoglycans (GAGs) are large polysaccharides with a repeating disaccharide pattern, e.g. hyaluronic acid, chondroitin sulphate and heparin. These molecules are highly negatively charged making them very hydrophilic. All GAGs, apart from hyaluronic acid, are sulphated and found as **proteoglycans** (linked to core proteins). GAGs and proteoglycans play several important roles in the body:

1. Their ability to take up water allows them to occupy large volumes. They make up the extracellular ground substance which fills the spaces between cells, providing resistance to compressive forces.
2. The aqueous nature of the gel formed by these molecules allows it to act as a molecular sieve regulating movement of molecules according to size and charge. This property is thought to be important in renal function. However nutrients, metabolites and signalling molecules can still diffuse freely through it.
3. GAGs and proteoglycans can bind to extracellular enzymes such as proteinases and to signalling molecules, e.g. growth factors and cytokines. This means that they can control both the distribution and the activity of these molecules.

There are more than 25 genes that encode proteins capable of forming proteoglycans. Structurally, the proteoglycans can be divided into two groups.

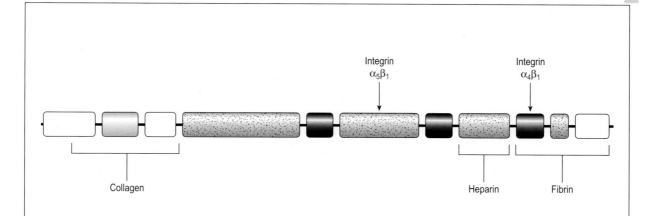

Fig. 11.3 A fibronectin monomer. Fibronectin is composed of many homologous repeating subunits. Regions of type I (open boxes), type II (grey boxes) and type III (stippled boxes) fibronectin repeats are shown. The three regions where alternative splicing can occur are indicated by black boxes. Binding sites for integrins and regions of the molecule responsible for binding to collagen, heparin and fibrin are indicated.

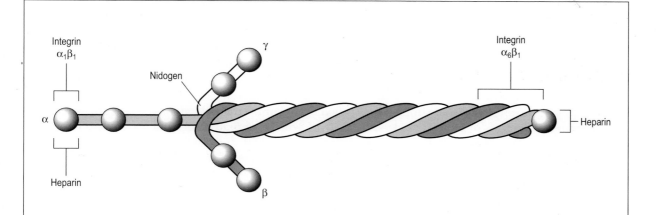

Fig. 11.4 The heterotrimeric structure of laminin-1. Globular domains are represented as circles. Proposed binding sites for integrins, nidogen (enactin) and heparin/heparan sulphate are indicated. Binding of laminin to perlecan (important in basal laminae) and α-dystroglycan is probably mediated through heparan sulphate.

Small leucine-rich proteoglycans (SLRPs)

These molecules are characterized by alternating hydrophobic and hydrophilic amino acids and feature multiple repeated motifs that contain conserved leucine residues. The most widely studied SLRP is decorin (Fig. 11.5), which binds to collagen (type I and II) and appears to have a role in controlling fibril formation: a decrease in fibril-associated decorin leads to the formation of thicker fibres of collagen. Decorin also has a potentially important role in inhibiting cell proliferation through its ability to bind and inactivate transforming growth factor beta (TGFβ).

Modular proteoglycans

The second group of proteoglycans are referred to as modular proteoglycans. Members of the group have many protein domains that share homology with a variety of cell surface and extracellular proteins, for example, immunoglobulin repeats, lectins (carbohydrate-binding proteins), epidermal growth factor (EGF), complement regulatory proteins and laminin. The modular proteoglycans include aggrecan, whose large numbers of GAG chains contribute to gel formation, and perlecan (Fig. 11.6). Perlecan, which is the principal heparan sulphate proteoglycan of the basement membrane, interacts with laminin and is deposited in embryonic ECM at an early stage of development. The heparan sulphate chains of perlecan bind a variety of growth factors and cytokines, storing them ready for release. It is thought that the release of growth factors from perlecan and other proteoglycans by platelet proteinases may play an important role in the response of tissues to injury. Modular proteoglycans are also important in the development of the nervous system, modulating the homophilic interactions of NCAM and acting as barriers to axonal outgrowth, thus determining the path of migrating axons.

Basal laminae

In addition to providing tensile strength, elasticity and resistance to compressive forces, ECM components combine to form strong sheets called **basal laminae**. Basal laminae, which are formed from mesh-like mats of type IV collagen interwoven with other matrix constituents, such as laminin, perlecan and nidogen (which links laminin to type IV collagen), are found in a variety of locations. In the kidney they play a filtering role, lying between epithelial and endothelial layers in the glomerulus. Basal laminae are also found underneath epithelial sheets, where they determine cell polarity and influence cell growth and differentiation, and surrounding muscle cells, where they are vital for the proper organization of neuromuscular junctions.

Defects in ECM proteins (particularly the collagens) give rise to several serious inherited diseases. Some examples are shown in Table 11.2.

Control of the ECM

Like all components, the amount of extracellular matrix in a tissue is a function of the balance between synthesis and degradation. Although ECM, having a structural role, might be considered rather fixed, local turnover is necessary to permit cell migration, e.g. infiltration of neutrophils at a site of injury or infection, or during tissue remodelling. The ability to penetrate the ECM and basal laminae is an important characteristic of metastatic tumour cells as they spread to remote sites. Matrix proteins such as collagen and laminin are degraded by zinc containing **metalloproteinases** (MMPs) and **serine proteinases** (e.g. elastase and cathepsins). Obviously such potentially destructive enzymes must be tightly regulated so that their action is limited. This is achieved in part by controlling transcription, but also by secreting MMPs as inactive precursors (**zymogens**), requiring activation by proteolytic cleavage. This activation step is probably mostly carried out by a distinct group of MMPs, the membrane-type or MT-metalloproteinases, which have a transmembrane domain anchoring them to the surface of the producing cells. A further level of control is provided by the production of specific inhibitors, the **tissue inhibitors of metalloproteinases** (TIMPS).

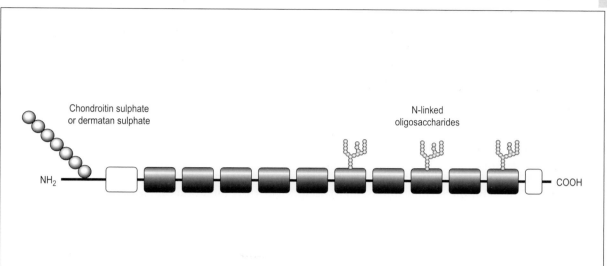

Fig. 11.5 Schematic diagram of the small leucine rich proteoglycan decorin. Open boxes indicate cysteine-rich regions, and filled boxes leucine-rich repeats.

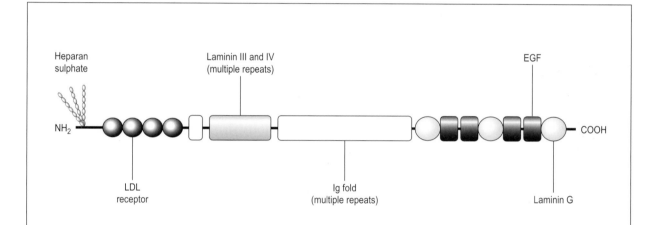

Fig. 11.6 Simplified diagram of the modular proteoglycan perlecan. Perlecan carries repeated sequences homologous to the low density lipoprotein (LDL) receptor, laminin domains III, IV and G, the immunoglobulin (Ig) fold and epidermal growth factor (EGF).

Matrix component	Disease	Symptoms
Collagen (type I)	Osteogenesis imperfecta	Weak bones – frequent fractures, deafness
Collagen (type II)	Chondroplasia	Abnormal cartilage, bone and joint deformities
Collagen (type III)[a]	Ehlers–Danlos syndrome	Fragile blood vessels, hyperelastic skin, lax joints
Collagen (type IV)	Alport syndrome	Nephritis leading to renal failure, deafness
Fibrillin[b]	Marfan syndrome	Long limbs, poor eyesight, aortic dilatation leading to aneurysm
Merosin (laminin α_2)	Congenital muscular dystrophy	Severe muscle wasting

Table 11.2 Inherited disorders resulting from deficiencies in extracellular matrix proteins. [a]Patients also show changes in fibronectin splicing, although these are probably secondary. [b]Fibrillin, which is defective in patients with Marfan's syndrome, is a vital component of microfibrils that are associated with elastin in elastic fibres

Further reading

Mercurio A M 1995 Laminin receptors: achieving specificity through co-operation. Trends in Cell Biology 5: 419–423

Iozzo R V, Murdoch A D 1996 Proteoglycans of the extracellular environment: clues from the gene and protein side offer novel perspectives in molecular diversity and function. FASEB Journal 10: 598–614

Revision questions

1. The fibronectin transcript exhibits alternate splicing. How might this alter the activities of the final protein?

2. How can proteoglycans influence cell growth and tissue repair?

3. What roles do metalloproteinases play in cell migration?

4. Why are the non-helical regions of fibrillar procollagens retained until after the molecules have left the cell?

Answers to revision questions

1. The inclusion or exclusion of particular binding domains may produce fibronectin molecules with different specificities.

2. The heparan sulphate chains of proteoglycans, such as perlecan, bind a variety of growth factors and cytokines, storing them ready for release. These growth factors can be released by platelet proteinases in response to injury.

3. Metalloproteinases degrade collagen and laminin thus clearing a path for migratory cells and may, in addition, uncover binding sites for cell adhesion molecules.

4. To prevent polymerization occurring within the cell. In addition to the potential for damage to the cell, polymerized collagen would be difficult to export.

Cell locomotion is important for a range of processes including immunological cell infiltration of tissues in inflammation and immunity, fertilization, embryological development, and tissue repair and turnover. The mechanisms responsible for cell movements can also be important for propelling extracellular materials past cells in processes such as wound healing. Three types of cell motion can be described: **random motion**; **chemokinesis**, a non-directional increase in cell movement in response to a chemical stimulus; and **chemotaxis**, the purposeful movement towards or away from a chemical stimulus.

Cilia and flagella in cell motility

One mechanism driving cell propulsion, particularly single cells such as spermatozoa, is the beating of a flagellum or cilia. When immobilized in tissues, such as epithelia, the beating of cilia then plays a role in the passage of extracellular materials past the cells, e.g. cilia in the bronchiolar epithelium beat to provide the outward driving force for removal of mucus and debris from the lungs.

Cell movements over the substratum

Cells may crawl over their substratum in a jerky movement by about a millimeter or so a day (Fig. 12.1). Forward-directed flattened protrusions are extended from the leading edge and adhere to the substrate through new **adhesion plaques**, allowing the body of the cell to be drawn forward. In cell culture, the dorsal surface of flattened fibroblasts becomes characteristically ruffled at and behind the leading edge, **leading lamella** or **lamellipodium** of the cell (Fig 12.2). The membrane 'ruffles', formed at sites of rapid actin polymerization, move backwards away from the lamellipodium. Dorsal membrane ruffling in culture may simply reflect a lack of adhesion to this cell surface. Similar retrograde movement of structures on the 'ventral' surface may provide the backwards driving or tractive force for movement of the leading edge.

Paradoxically, as the cell moves forwards there is a retrograde movement of larger membrane constituents away from the leading edge. A 'raking' mechanism has been proposed in which larger molecules become associated with transmembranous adhesion proteins, which in turn are linked to backward-moving actin microfilaments in the advancing tip of the lamellipodium (Fig. 12.3). The microfilaments are orientated with their positive, growing ends towards the leading edge such that treadmilling of the filaments results in an extension of the lamellipodium in the forward direction and a retrograde motion of the adhesion proteins that are fixed to the actin microfilaments. Inhibition of actin filament polymerization at the growing end due to the proximity of the lamellipodial membrane may be prevented simply by thermal motion of the filament end. Alternatively, it has been proposed that an osmotic swelling mechanism at the leading edge could provide the space for continued actin polymerization.

To restore membrane macromolecules and lipid that may have been removed by the 'raking' activity at the lamellipodium membrane, vesicles derived from the Golgi apparatus fuse with the lamellipodial membrane, reincorporating new and recycled proteins and lipid at the leading edge (Fig. 12.4). In some, but not all cells, vesicles from the Golgi apparatus are directed by microtubules. Even before lamellipodia are formed, the microtubule-organizing centre (MTOC) is orientated such that the vesicles from the Golgi are directed to the leading edge, thereby polarizing the cell.

The direction of chemotactic cell migration is determined by membrane receptors for chemotactic stimuli. How these messages are translated into intracellular events remains unknown. Indeed, because of the lability of locomotor mechanisms and the complexity of cellular processes involved, a complete description of cell locomotion remains to be elucidated.

Further reading

Harris A K 1994 Locomotion of tissue culture cells considered in relation to ameboid locomotion. International Review of Cytology 150: 35–69

Lauffenburger D A, Horwitz A F 1996 Cell-migration – a physically integrated molecular process. Cell 84: 359–369

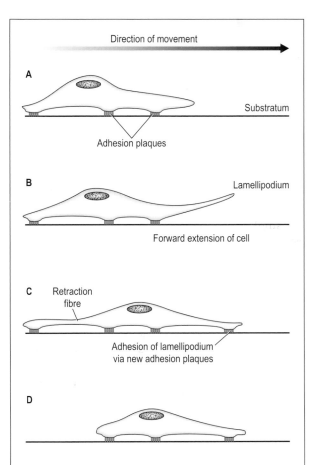

Fig. 12.1 Schematic diagram of fibroblast locomotion over a substratum surface. (**A**) The fibroblast is attached to the substratum via adhesion plaques. (**B**) Lamellipodia extend from the leading edge of the cell and (**C**) attach to the substratum via new adhesion plaques. Cellular materials are withdrawn from the tail of the cell along actin microfilaments by an ATP-dependent mechanism. This results in cell narrowing to form **retraction fibres** (**D**). The tail detaches and the remaining contents are drawn forward into the cell. Proteases secreted near adhesion plaques also contribute to detachment of trailing regions, e.g. urokinase.

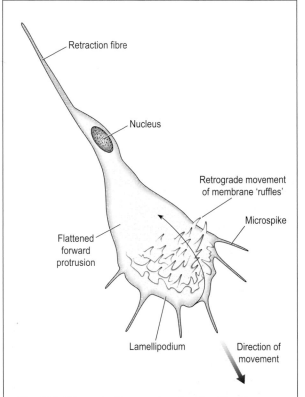

Fig. 12.2 Schematic diagram of a migrating fibroblast showing the retrograde movement of 'ruffles' over the 'dorsal' surface.

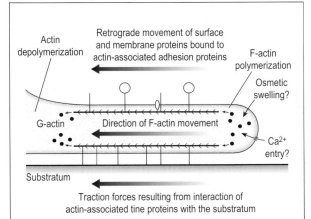

Fig. 12.3 Relationship between actin microfilament 'treadmilling', membrane 'raking' and surface transport and tractive forces in an extending lamellipodium. Osmotic swelling and/or Ca^{2+} entry in the lamellipodium may be required to facilitate actin filament extension.

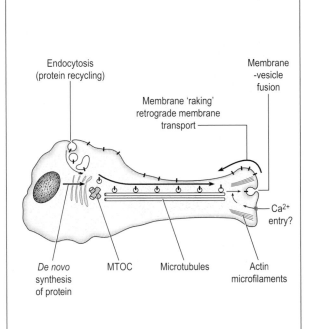

Fig. 12.4 Schematic diagram of membrane vesicle trafficking in migrating cells. Fusion of exocytotic vesicles at the lamellipodium replenishes membrane components removed by membrane 'raking' either by recycling them or by delivering newly synthesized components. MTOC, microtubule-organizing centre.

Cell growth, cell division and the cell cycle

Cell division is important for growth, development, repair and replacement of dead cells. In an organism made up of multiple cell types and tissues, it is most important that cell proliferation is tightly regulated. The consequence of a loss of control in a cell is cancer.

The cell cycle

Stages of the cell cycle

The process of cell division is cyclical and unidirectional (Fig. 13.1). The period between successive cell divisions is termed the **interphase**. Interphase begins with a period of rapid biosynthesis and cell growth, G_1 **(gap) phase**, to provide cellular constituents for a second new cell. This phase of the cell cycle is the most variable in duration (minutes to months). In non-dividing tissues, cells withdraw from the cell cycle into a **resting state (G_0)**, but can re-enter G_1 upon stimulation. After G_1, the cell moves into **S phase** when the complete genomic DNA is duplicated. After S phase a second gap phase, G_2 **phase**, prepares the cell for the **M phase** where **mitosis**, the division of nuclear material, and **cytokinesis**, the process of cytoplasmic division, occur such that the two daughter cells each receive a complete copy of the genomic DNA.

G_0 to G_1 transition (mitogenesis)

Proliferation of quiescent cells (G_0) can be induced by **mitogens** in a cell-type-specific manner. Mitogens include growth factors, hormones and cell contact. Signalling pathways activated by mitogens (Chapter 7) lead to the expression of responsive genes and the progression of the cell through G_1 and past a '**restriction point**' (mammalian cells) or **START** (yeast), where the cell becomes committed to a complete division cycle. Once past the restriction point, cells no longer require the presence of growth factors and are unresponsive to anti-mitogenic signals, such as transforming growth factor β (TGFβ). Protein expression induced by mitogens includes some cyclins (see below), sequence-specific transcription factors (e.g. by *myc*, *fos*, *jun* genes), DNA-binding receptors and other proteins.

Regulation of the cell cycle

Progression through the cell cycle is controlled at three '**checkpoints**' between the stages of the cycle: **restriction point**, **mitosis entry** and **mitosis exit**. These monitor, respectively, the availability of nutrients/growth factors, DNA replication/damage and assembly of the mitotic spindle. Transition between stages is triggered by increased activity of specific **cyclin-dependent protein kinases (CDK)** (Fig. 13.2). Each CDK is presumed to phosphorylate, and thereby modulate the activity of, a subset of cellular target proteins specific for progression through individual transitions within the cell cycle. For example, the S-phase CDK (CDK2/cyclin D, E or A) may phosphorylate proteins involved in DNA replication, while **mitosis-promoting factor (MPF)** (Cdc2 (CDK1)/cyclin B) may phosphorylate proteins during mitosis such as the nuclear lamins, histones and cytoskeletal proteins involved in chromosome condensation, assembly of the mitotic spindle, dissolution of the nuclear membrane and cell detachment.

Control of cyclin-dependent protein kinase activity by cyclin expression

Levels of CDK proteins remain relatively constant throughout the cell cycle but their activity is regulated at different stages. CDKs are activated primarily by the binding of specific **cyclins**. The levels of the different cyclins rise and fall at different points in the cell cycle and produce temporal activation of their specific CDK (Fig. 13.3). For example, the synthesis of cyclin B is relatively constant and concentrations rise in a linear manner until a threshold is reached when Cdc2 is activated and the cell proceeds into mitosis. At mitosis the rate of cyclin B breakdown is accelerated and the stimulation of Cdc2 is terminated. The levels of other cyclins, e.g. E, are more closely controlled at the level of expression and mRNA for these species is only present during limited phases of the cell cycle.

CDKs are also subject to complex modulation in response to several intracellular signalling pathways. This serves to integrate intra- and extracellular signals reflecting nutritional status and intercellular communication. Whether or not a cell proceeds to the next stage of the cell cycle, therefore, depends on the integration of multiple factors at the level of the CDK.

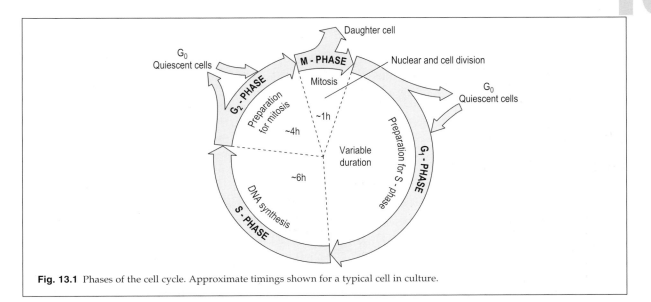

Fig. 13.1 Phases of the cell cycle. Approximate timings shown for a typical cell in culture.

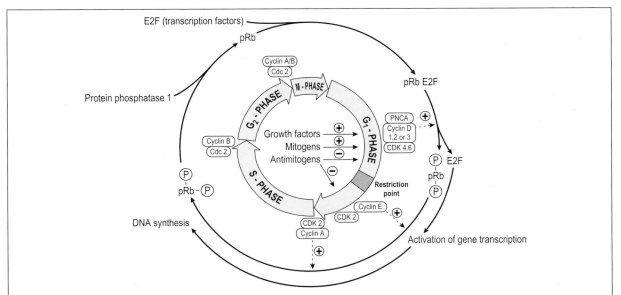

Fig. 13.2 Cyclin-dependent protein kinase (CDK, Cdc) and retinoblastoma tumour suppressor gene product (pRb) in the control of the cell cycle.

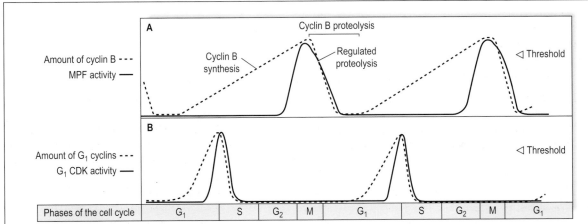

Fig. 13.3 Activation of cyclin-dependent protein kinase (CDK, Cdc) activity during the cell cycle by cyclins. Note that the amount of CDK is relatively constant throughout the cell cycle. CDK activity is regulated by the synthesis and breakdown of the appropriate cyclins.

Tumour suppressor genes regulate the passage into S phase

Most of the substrates for CDKs remain unknown. However, one mechanism at the G_1–S checkpoint may involve the hyperphosphorylation of negative cell cycle regulators, such as the retinoblastoma tumour suppressor gene product (pRb), to overcome their suppression of passage from G_1 (see Fig. 13.2). In normal quiescent cells and early G_1, pRb is found in a hypophosphorylated form, which actively binds several cytoplasmic proteins. Phosphorylation of pRb by G_1 CDK (CDK2/cyclin D) results in the release of these proteins, including transcription factors of the E2F family, which go on to activate transcription of the S-phase genes. Therefore, in G_1, pRb appears to act as a cell cycle suppressor by binding members of the E2F transcription factor family. pRb is absent or inactive in retinoblastoma and several other tumours suggesting that, in its absence, passage through the G_1–S checkpoint goes unchecked (see below).

DNA replication in S phase

Replication against the 3′–5′ strand (Fig. 13.4). During S phase (6–8 h) each of the 46 chromatin chromosomes are replicated to form a sister chromatid joined to the original molecule through a structure called the **centromere**. DNA replication commences at specific **origin of replication sites** with ATP-dependent unwinding of the chromatin structure by **DNA helicase** to form sites at which a priming **RNA polymerase** can bind. **DNA topoisomerase** also acts to break and rejoin the unwound strands to prevent tangling of the structure due to supercoiling. **Single-stranded DNA binding protein** binds to the unwound strands to protect them from degradation before DNA duplication begins. Initiation requires the 5′–3′ synthesis of a small RNA fragment (10–20 nucleotides) against the template strand (**leading strand**) reading in the 3′–5′ direction. This is catalysed by specific **RNA polymerases** or **primases**, which do not require priming oligonucleotides. Using the RNA fragment as primer, **DNA polymerase III** then catalyses the efficient incorporation of base-paired nucleotides against the leading strand and the elongation reaction which forms the sister chain in the 5′–3′ polarity. Thus, at each origin of replication site two DNA polymerase complexes can bind and two **replication forks** are generated, which move away from each other as synthesis proceeds (Fig. 13.5).

Replication against the 5′–3′ strand (Fig. 13.4). As DNA polymerase does not catalyse synthesis in the 3′–5′ direction, synthesis against the other parental strand (5′–3′ **lagging strand**) must occur in the opposite direction. DNA duplication on the lagging strand is by a different discontinuous mechanism and produces short fragments (~1000 nucleotides) of new DNA, termed **Okazaki fragments**. As on the leading strand, duplication is initiated by synthesis of an RNA primer, which directs synthesis of DNA against the lagging strand by **DNA polymerase III**. This occurs until the polymerase meets the initiating RNA primer of the preceding segment of DNA sequence resulting in an Okazaki fragment. It has been proposed that dimeric DNA polymerase acts on a looped DNA structure at each replication fork so that DNA synthesis occurs on both strands essentially simultaneously (Fig. 13.6). To complete the new DNA strand generated against the lagging strand, the short sections of RNA are removed by a **5′–3′ RNase H**. **DNA polymerase I** completes the DNA strand in the gap and adjacent DNA fragments are then joined by a **DNA ligase** driven by hydrolysis of ATP or NAD⁺ (some prokaryotes).

✎ DNA replication inhibitors in cancer therapy

Synthesis of nucleotides to sustain DNA synthesis in S phase is clearly most important. Disruption of the supply of any of the four nucleotides leads to interruption of the cell cycle in S phase. This is the basis of anti-cancer therapies using drugs such as 5-fluorouracil and methoxytrexate, which block the synthesis of dTTP. Such treatments are non-specific and target rapidly dividing cells in particular, which includes tumour cells. Other rapidly dividing tissues such as progenitor blood cells, gut epithelium, skin and hair follicles are also affected and these effects underlie the major unwanted effects of these drugs of anaemia, sickness and hair loss. In particular, patients become immunosuppressed owing to drug-induced neutropenia and may become platelet-depleted leading to bruising and increased risk of haemorrhage.

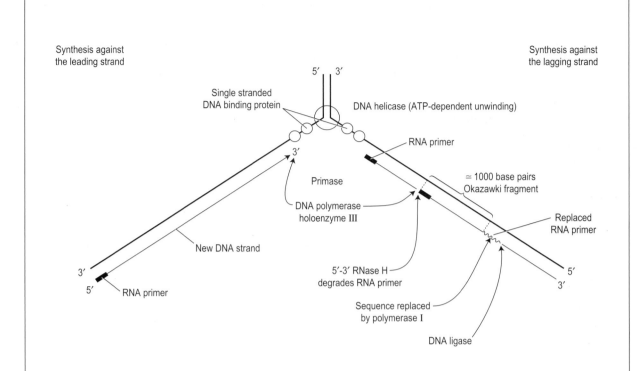

Synthesis against
the leading strand

Synthesis against
the lagging strand

Single stranded
DNA binding protein

DNA helicase (ATP-dependent unwinding)

5′ 3′

RNA primer

Primase

3′

New DNA strand

DNA polymerase
holoenzyme III

≃ 1000 base pairs
Okazawki fragment

Replaced
RNA primer

3′

5′   RNA primer

5′-3′ RNase H
degrades RNA primer

5′

3′

Sequence replaced
by polymerase I

DNA ligase

Fig. 13.4 DNA replication against leading and lagging DNA strands at the replication fork. Once formed, the sister DNA strands are repackaged into nucleosomes and higher order structures before cell division. Old histones associate with the parent strands but the provision of histones for the packing of sister chromatids is one reason why protein synthesis is increased during S phase. Multiple copies of each histone gene ensures that histone synthesis keeps pace with demand for chromatin packing during S phase. Additional proteins must associate following DNA duplication to prevent further duplications before cell division.

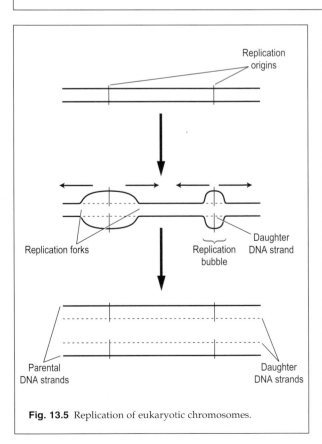

Replication
origins

Replication forks

Replication
bubble

Daughter
DNA strand

Parental
DNA strands

Daughter
DNA strands

Fig. 13.5 Replication of eukaryotic chromosomes.

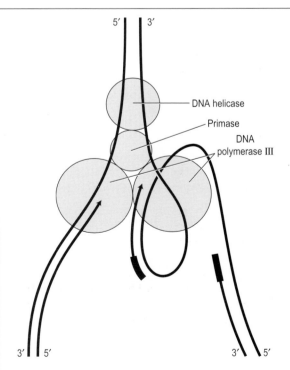

5′ 3′

DNA helicase

Primase

DNA
polymerase III

3′ 5′

3′ 5′

Fig. 13.6 Looping of the lagging strand may permit the simultaneous synthesis of DNA against both template DNA strands by dimeric DNA polymerase.

151

Replicons

To ensure that the whole genome is replicated within the short time period of S phase, multiple replication forks are activated in clusters (up to 100) on each chromosome. Replication forks moving in opposite directions from adjacent origin of replication sites meet eventually over **termination sites** and the adjacent segments of new DNA are ligated. The length of DNA produced between two origins is approximately the same as that required by one loop of the chromatin structure or a single gene and is termed a **replicon** (up to 300 000 base pairs).

Cell cycle arrest

The cell cycle may be arrested at two points (G_1–S and G_2–M) as a result of DNA damage. Mechanisms of cell cycle arrest are not well characterized but appear often to involve inhibition of CDKs as part of their action (Fig. 13.7). For example, the tumour suppressor gene product p53 is important in arresting the cell cycle at G_1 and may stimulate DNA repair indirectly. Expression of p53 is normally low but is increased dramatically when cell DNA is damaged, leading to the suggestion that it is a 'guardian of the genome'.

DNA repair

Maintaining the integrity of the genetic information carried by the DNA of an organism is vital to survival. In addition to depurination (loss of a purine base) and deamination (loss of an amine group from a base), which occur spontaneously (5–10 000 and 100 times per genome per day, respectively), the cell must resist the effects of environmental agents such as chemical mutagens and physical forces (e.g. ultraviolet (UV) radiation, X-rays, cosmic radiation). Some damage is self-inflicted, the result of errors in replication, and there are specific mismatch repair enzymes that scan newly synthesized DNA replacing wrongly incorporated bases. Unrepaired damage can lead to mutation, loss of information and even block replication. As a consequence, cells express several enzymes whose task is to repair damaged DNA before it is replicated (Table 13.1). This task is approached in two ways. Simple lesions, such as those caused by alkylation of bases, may be reversed, whilst other lesions are removed and replaced with new DNA.

Reversal of damage

Alkylating agents such as nitrosoureas and nitrogen mustards add alkyl groups to guanine residues (and other bases to a lesser degree). These alkyl groups may be removed by alkyl transferase enzymes, thus reversing the damage.

Replacement of damaged bases

Deaminated bases are cleaved from the sugar–phosphate backbone by specific DNA glycosylases. The resulting apurinic or apyrimidinic sites (along with those produced by spontaneous depurination) are recognized by specific AP (apurinic or apyrimidinic) endonucleases which nick the sugar–phosphate backbone next to the AP site. The damaged base can then be removed by exonucleases, and new DNA synthesized by DNA polymerase using the undamaged strand as template (Fig. 13.8). The repair process is completed by DNA ligase, which seals the nick in the backbone. Larger lesions, such as the pyrimidine (cyclobutane) dimers produced by UV radiation, are corrected by excision repair, where a short stretch of the damaged strand is removed and replaced by new DNA.

Xeroderma pigmentosa

Dysfunction of the nucleotide excision repair process in humans leads to the rare disease **xeroderma pigmentosa**. Mutations in over seven different genes may contribute to this disease. These individuals are sensitive to UV radiation, which results in the accumulation of pyrimidine dimers in cells. As a result, severe skin lesions develop, including cancers.

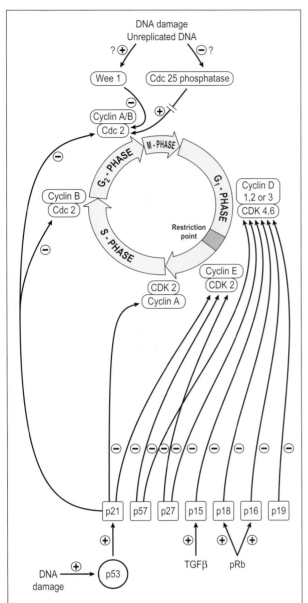

Fig. 13.7 Cell cycle arrest involves the inhibition of cyclin-dependent protein kinases (CDK, Cdc) by inhibitor proteins or phosphorylation. Cyclin-dependent protein kinase inhibitors (CKI) are shown in boxes. Wee 1, CDK kinase; p53, tumour suppressor gene; TGFβ, transforming growth factor β. Note: over-expression of cyclin D1 is associated with human parathyroid cancer and B cell lymphoma as a result of chromosome inversion and translocation, respectively.

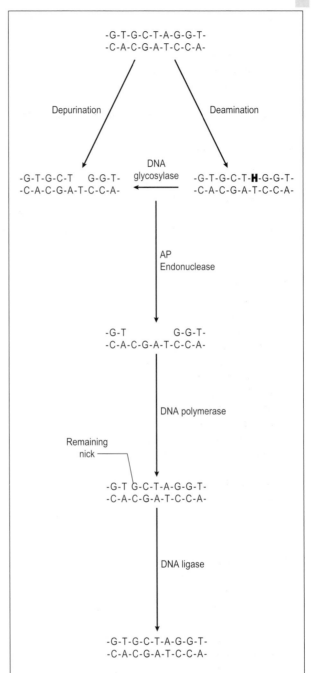

Fig. 13.8 DNA repair: excision of a damaged base and synthesis of new DNA.

Lesion	Causative agent	Consequence	Repair mechanism
Deamination	Spontaneous	Converts C to uracil (which pairs with A instead of G) and A to hypoxanthine (which pairs with C instead of T)	Base excision by glycosylase
Depurination	Spontaneous	Non-informative, can pair with any base	Nicking of backbone by AP endonucleases and repair synthesis
Alkylation	Alkylating agents e.g. nitrosoureas.	Altered pairing properties (dependent on specific lesion)	Removal of alkyl groups by alkyl transferases
Strand breaks	Ionizing radiation		Ligation (single-strand breaks) or recombination (double-strand breaks)
Cyclobutane dimers	UV radiation	Block replication	Excision repair

Table 13.1 DNA damage and DNA repair mechanisms

Mitosis

M phase is a continuous dynamic process in vivo but can be subdivided into five mitotic stages (nuclear division) followed by a sixth stage of cytokinesis (cytoplasmic division) (Fig. 13.9). Mitosis is necessarily a highly accurate process to ensure the correct segregation of sister chromosomes.

Prophase (Fig. 13.9A). As the cell moves from G_2 phase into prophase the sister chromatids, duplicated during interphase, begin to condense into well-defined chromosomal structures and the nucleolus is disassembled. In the cytoplasm the microtubular cytoskeletal network is also disassembled and reorganized on the surface of the nucleus to form the basis of the **mitotic spindle**. This structure is a bipolar arrangement of polar microtubules, which is capped at each end by a pair of centrioles or **mitotic centre** (the centriole pair is duplicated during S phase) from which astral microtubules radiate. During prophase the two asters, which begin lying side by side, are pushed away from each other by the growing bundles of polar microtubules forming the polar mitotic spindle.

Prometaphase (Fig. 13.9B). The disruption of the nuclear envelope into vesicular fragments signals the beginning of prometaphase. During this phase microtubules associate with specialized points of attachment in the pericentriolar material on either side of the centromeres of condensed chromosomes called **kinetochores**. With the dissolution of the nuclear envelope the kinetochore microtubules form initially random associations with the mitotic spindle and gradually orientate alongside the polar microtubular network. Then by a series of jerky movements the chromosomes are rearranged at right angles to the mitotic spindle (**metaphase plate**) so that the centromeres are aligned.

Metaphase (Fig. 13.9C). When the chromosomes are aligned at the centre of the mitotic spindle the cell is said to be in metaphase. Each chromosome is held in position at the metaphase plate by the kinetochore microtubules attached to the paired kinetochores. This phase appears as a period of relative inactivity during nuclear division and can last a relatively long time.

Anaphase (Fig. 13.9D). In anaphase the centromere splits in two, the paired kinetochores separate and the sister chromosomes migrate towards the opposite poles of the mitotic spindle. The kinetochore microtubules are seen to shorten as the chromosomes migrate towards the poles and at the same time the polar microtubules elongate increasing the separation between the poles of the spindle. Chromosomes are, therefore, pulled towards the mitotic poles while the poles themselves are pushed apart. This phase often starts abruptly and lasts only a few minutes.

Telophase (Fig. 13.9E). Telophase marks the end of nuclear division. The kinetochore microtubules disassemble completely and the polar microtubules elongate still further before the mitotic spindle finally dissociates at the end of nuclear division. During this phase the nuclear membrane reforms, the chromosomes begin to decondense into the dispersed chromatin structure and nucleoli begin to reform in the daughter nuclei.

Cytokinesis (Fig. 13.9F). The division of the cytoplasm is achieved by the formation of an actin microfilament ring under the plasma membrane at right angles to the mitotic spindle in the region of the cell corresponding to the position of the metaphase plate. Contraction of this structure commences usually in late anaphase to form a **cleavage furrow**. The cleavage furrow deepens progressively until the opposing edges meet and membrane fusion results in the completed division of the two daughter cells. Formation of the cleavage furrow may be arrested for a while if it meets residual mitotic spindle structures to form a **midbody**.

The result of mitotic cell division is the production of two daughter cells that contain a complete copy of the genome of the parent cell.

Inhibitors of mitosis in cancer therapy

Treatment of mitotic cells with anti-mitotic, anti-cancer drugs such as **colchicine, vinblastine** and **vincristine**, which disrupt microtubule assembly, causes the dissappearance of the mitotic spindle and blocks the cells in metaphase. By contrast, **taxol** causes mitotic arrest by stabilizing the mitotic spindle.

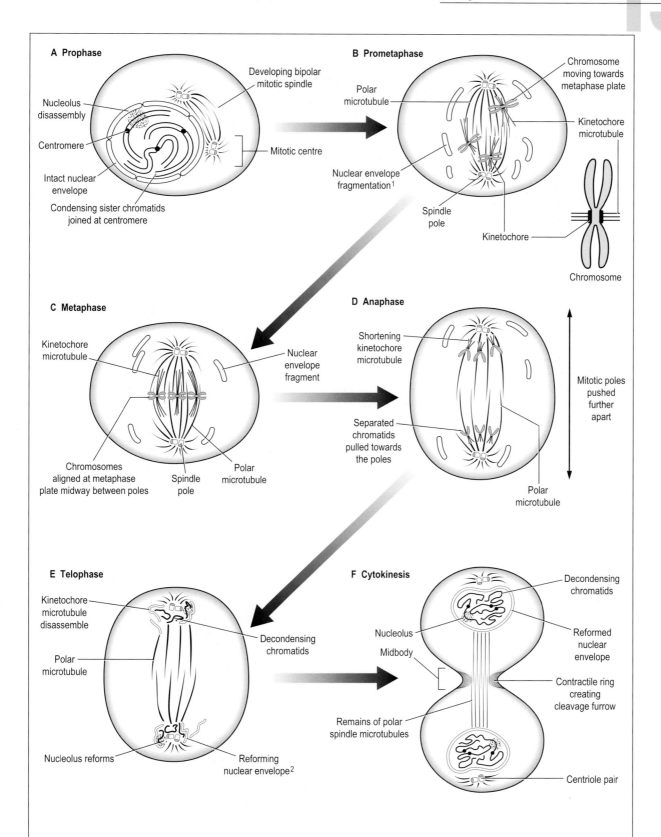

Fig. 13.9 The six stages of mitotic cell division. 1 — nuclear envelope disintegration is accompanied by phosphorylation and resulting dissociation of the nuclear microfilament network. B lamin remains associated with residual nuclear membrane fragments while lamins A and C are released into the cytoplasm. 2 — in telophase, a phospholamin phosphatase on the chromatin dephosphorylates lamins A, B and C resulting in the repolymerization of the neurofilament network centred on the membrane-associated lamin B. This draws nuclear membrane vesicles into a position where they can fuse to reform the nuclear envelope.

Meiosis

Meiosis is a specialized form of cell division that produces four genetically distinct haploid cells (that contain only a single copy of each chromosome) from a diploid progenitor cell (containing two copies of each chromosome). This reductive form of cell division is found only in gamete production, in oogenesis and spermatogenesis. There are many similarities to mitotic cell division but also some important differences. Unlike mitosis, meiosis requires two rounds of cell division. The first round generates genetic variation and the second round produces haploid cells (Fig. 13.10). As in mitosis, meiosis can be divided into several stages.

Interphase. Before the first meiotic cell division the chromatin of the diploid parental cell is replicated to form sister chromatids joined at the centromere.

Prophase I. On entering the first round of division the sister chromatids, which remain associated (**bivalents**), condense into long thin strands stabilized by a central protein axis. As prophase continues, homologous chromosomes form closely associated pairs, **synapses**, along their entire length bringing equivalent genes into apposition. The condensing structure forms a ladder-like proteinaceous axis from the two contributing chromosomes against which the chromatids are aligned, termed the **synaptonemal complex**. When the synapsis is complete, a period of **recombination** or **crossing-over** occurs (pachytene) where segments of paired maternal and paternal DNA can be exchanged between homologous chromosomes, resulting in increased genetic variation in the germ cell lines. On average two to three crossing-over events occur per pair of chromosomes. The two homologous chromosomes in a bivalent then decondense but as they move away from each other they remain associated at points at which cross-over events have taken place, **chiasmata**. RNA synthesis may occur against the unravelling chromatids. This is important for the production of storage material during the development of **oocytes** (eggs). In the late part of this phase (diakenesis), the chromosomes condense and each bivalent is observed to contain four chromatids, with sister chromatids joined at the centromere and non-sister chromatids joined at the chiasmata. The nuclear envelope breaks down releasing the condensed chromosomes to interact with the completed spindle structure. Prophase I is the longest stage in meiotic cell division and completion of division I and the whole of division II may only take 10% of the time spent in prophase I.

Metaphase I. In metaphase I the synaptic pairs of chromosomes move to the equator of the cell and orientate at right angles to the spindle. Although non-identical, the X and Y sex chromosomes also pair owing to a region of similarity within their structure.

Anaphase I. Unlike the mitotic anaphase, the sister chromatids remain associated by the centromeres. Instead, the homologous synaptic pairs separate towards opposite poles of the spindle. The result of the first nuclear division is two diploid cells that are genetically distinct because of the independent assortment of parental chromosomes and recombination events.

The second meiotic division. The interphase between the first and second meiotic cell divisions does not involve DNA replication, and differs therefore from the first meiotic division and mitosis. In other ways the second meiotic cell division is analogous to mitosis. The sister chromatids separate at their centromeres during anaphase II and segregate to the opposite spindle pole. The result of meiotic cell division is the production of four cells that contain non-identical haploid copies of the genome (Fig. 13.10).

Down's syndrome

Down's syndrome, which arises from an extra copy of chromosome 21, develops during meiosis because of the failure of this chromosome to separate during meiosis I/II.

Genetic variation arises in meiosis

Assuming no recombination, the number of possible different combinations of chromosomes in gametes after independent assortment in humans would be 2^n (where n = number of chromosomes), i.e. 2^{23} or $\sim 8.4 \times 10^6$. The actual number of different combinations is much greater than this because of cross-over events during recombination in prophase I.

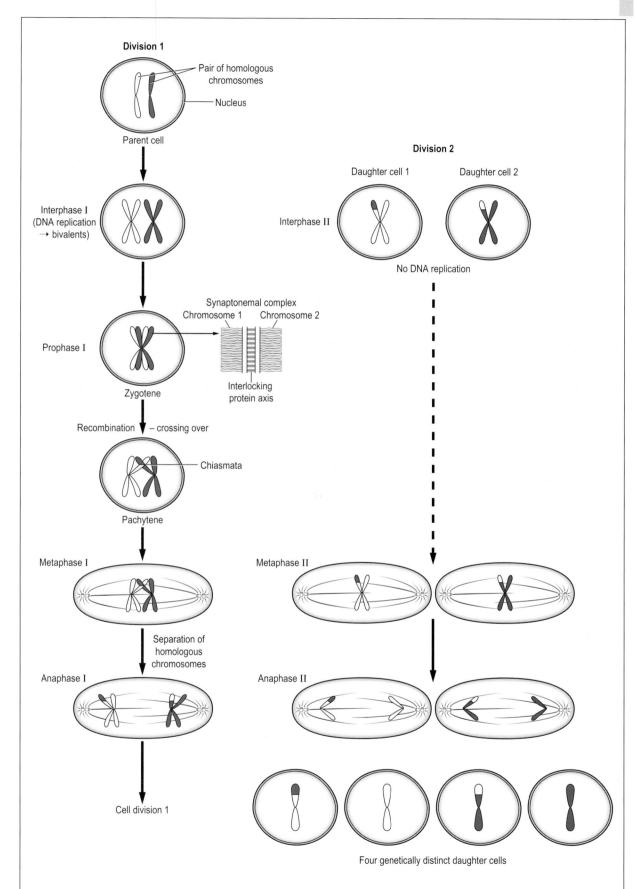

Fig. 13.10 Schematic summary of the first and second cell divisions of meiosis. Events are illustrated for one homologous chromosome pair only.

Gametes

Spermatogenesis (Fig. 13.11). In male mammals the four haploid cells produced by meiosis go on to differentiate into spermatozoa. The cytoplasm is reduced and the nucleus condensed and a motile flagellum is assembled to facilitate swimming.

Oogenesis. In females, meiosis is halted in prophase I to allow yolk production (Fig. 13.11). The first meiotic cell division is asymmetrical producing a secondary oocyte and a polar body much depleted in cytoplasmic constituents. This polar body is one of two small cells formed during meiotic divisions that serve as 'carriers' for extra chromosomes that the egg/zygote eliminates. The secondary oocyte passes into the second meiotic division to be arrested again at metaphase II. On maturation and release of the ovarian follicle the secondary oocyte remains in its arrested form. The second meiotic division is only completed when stimulated by the cellular events of fertilization. A further asymmetrical cell division occurs so that most of the cytoplasmic constituents are segregated into a single oocyte and a further polar body is formed. Only after meiosis is completed in the oocyte does mixing of the parental haploid genomes occur to form the zygote nucleus. The diploid polar bodies from the first division can also undergo a second meiotic cell division to produce two further haploid polar bodies. The result of meiosis in the female is one well-nourished haploid oocyte and three haploid polar bodies that are allowed to degenerate.

Fertilization

The fusion of egg and sperm at fertilization and the mixing of their haploid genomes restores the diploid genotype. As the sperm swim through the female reproductive tract they undergo an unknown process of **capacitation**, which permits them to fuse with an oocyte. Fusion begins via species-specific interactions with glycoproteins in the zona pellucida of the oocyte (Fig. 13.12A). A massive influx of Ca^{2+} is triggered in the **acrosome reaction**, which induces the release of hydrolytic enzymes from the acrosome vesicle of the sperm that digest the zona pellucida and allow the sperm to penetrate to the plasma membrane of the oocyte (Fig. 13.12B). Polymerization of actin in the sperm head results in an extension of an **acrosomal process** and when the sperm and oocyte plasma membranes meet they fuse (Fig. 13.12C). Fusion stimulates the immediate release of cortical granules from the oocyte containing enzymes that modify the zona pellucida to prevent penetration of further sperm, the entry of the sperm nucleus and a dramatic rise in $[Ca^{2+}]_i$ from the release of intracellular Ca^{2+} stores (Fig. 13.12D). This change stimulates the progression of meiosis from metaphase II in the secondary oocyte while the male chromosomes remain isolated within a pronucleus. Mixing of the maternal and paternal chromosomes in the zygote first occurs during the metaphase of the first mitotic division.

> ### Assisted conception
>
> Several methods of assisted conception have been developed for the treatment of infertility. In gamete intrafallopian transfer (GIFT), ova are collected and delivered to the oviduct laparoscopically. Partner or donor sperm is delivered at the same time and fertilization takes place in the fallopian tube. This procedure can be used where ovulation is impaired, for moderate sperm dysfunction or where there are problems with sperm transport in the female tract. Fertilization may also be achieved in vitro by mixing ova and sperm in a test tube. In this case only fertilized ova are selected for replacement and ova containing three or more pronuclei are discarded as this indicates fusion with two or more sperm. In vitro fertilization is indicated particularly when fallopian tubes are blocked. In cases of severe sperm dysfunction, fertilization may be achieved by intracytoplasmic sperm injection (ICSI). In this technique a single sperm is injected directly into an ovum selected to be in metaphase II. Interestingly, the acrosome reaction is bypassed by this procedure but injected ova still develop into normal zygotes. In some cases of severe male infertility, e.g. round-headed sperm (globozospermia), fertilization does not occur at high frequency even after ICSI, suggesting that additional factors are provided by the sperm to permit fertilization. It is also worth consideration that, although ICSI presents the only opportunity for conception to some infertile males, genetic defects in sperm production will be passed on to the next generation.

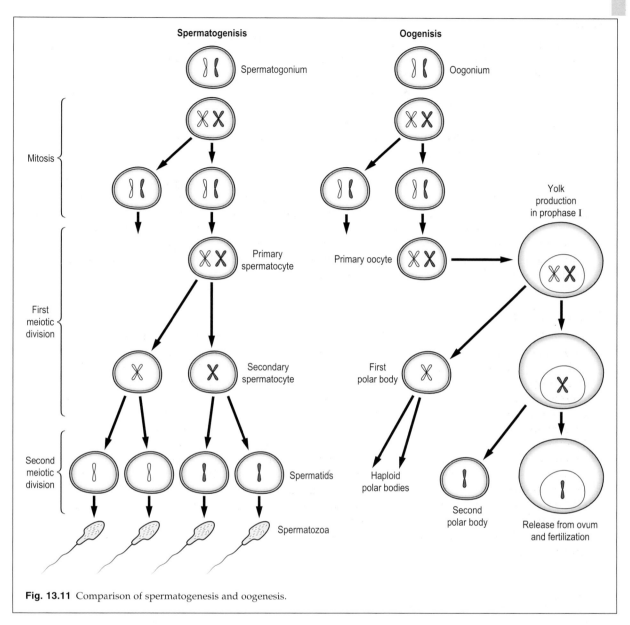

Fig. 13.11 Comparison of spermatogenesis and oogenesis.

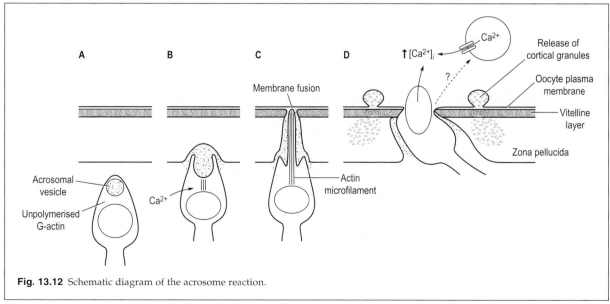

Fig. 13.12 Schematic diagram of the acrosome reaction.

Cancer

A cancer is an uncontrolled growth and division of cells that have escaped the normal regulatory mechanisms of the cell cycle. Cancerous or **tumour** or **neoplastic** cells are said to be transformed. Transformed cells characteristically continue to divide under conditions in which normal cells would become quiescent, i.e. when nutrients or growth factors are depleted from the medium. In cell culture the cytoskeleton fails to organize correctly and the cells assume a typically rounded appearance and no longer require attachment to substrate to grow. This leads to cells overgrowing each other in culture dishes, unlike normal cells where the division is arrested when a confluent monolayer is formed in the dish (Fig. 13.13). A cancer is said to be **benign** when the growth is localized to the site of origin within a tissue, with no invasion, and **malignant** when the tumour cells can invade into the surrounding tissue and vasculature, spread to distant sites and grow there forming secondary tumours (**metastasis**).

Tumourigenesis: the somatic cell theory of cancer

Cancers arise because of mutations in the genome of somatic cells as a result of inaccuracies in gene replication or chromosomal rearrangement at mitosis (Fig. 13.14). If a result of the mutation is loss of control of cell growth and division, the mutant cell divides more rapidly than the surrounding tissue to form a clone of daughter tumour cells. Tumourigenesis is complex and requires more than one somatic mutation before full transformation of the cell occurs (Fig. 13.15). Such a multistage process may occur over a period of years with contributory mutations being accumulated over many generations of the cell. Although the origin of cancer is genetic, it is not usually a hereditary disease. It is noteworthy that some rare familial predispositions to cancer are known. The somatic cell theory explains why cancers are not seen often in young people and why the incidence of cancer increases with age in the population.

Tumourigenic mutations most often arise because of inaccuracies in DNA replication, hereditary deficiencies in DNA repair and exposure to radiation or chemical **carcinogens**. Radiation (X-rays, γ-rays and UV light) may induce tumourigenic mutations by direct damage of the DNA or indirectly as a result of errors arising during subsequent DNA repair by the cell. The mutagenic action of many carcinogens is not known but some act by intercalating in double-stranded DNA and disrupting normal structure, thereby affecting DNA replication. Carcinogens may themselves be **mutagens** or processed in the liver into an active mutagenic form.

Viruses and tumourigenesis

Viral infection of cells is associated with several human cancers. One group of RNA viruses (single-stranded, diploid) and five groups of DNA viruses (all double-stranded) have been implicated. Association of RNA tumour viruses (retroviruses) with carcinogenesis in animals is well established but in humans most of the evidence implicating viral transformation is based on epidemiological studies. All of the tumour viruses insert their genome into that of the host for replication and thereafter are reproduced in daughter cells. Tumourigenesis results either from the disruption of the structure and/or expression of a local host cell gene or **proto-oncogene**, a process known as **insertional mutagenesis**, or from the expression of virally encoded genes, **oncogenes**, which are responsible directly for the transformation of the cell.

Viruses and human cancers

Examples of viral associations with human cancers include Epstein-Barr virus with Burkitt's lymphoma and nasopharyngeal cancer, hepatitis B with liver cancer, human immunodeficiency viruses with leukaemia and lymphoma and papillomaviruses, together with chemical carcinogens, with anogenital and some upper airway cancers.

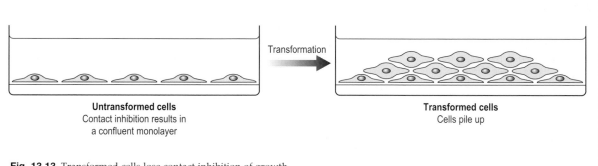

Fig. 13.13 Transformed cells lose contact inhibition of growth.

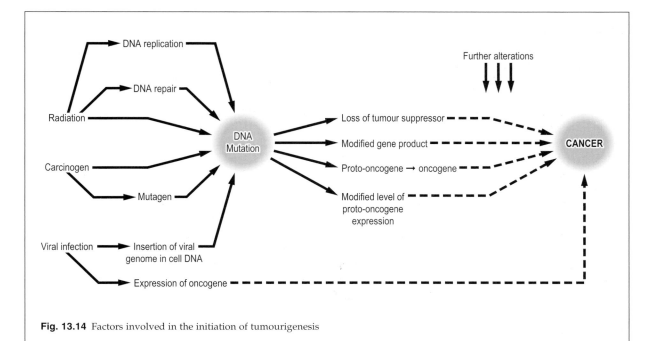

Fig. 13.14 Factors involved in the initiation of tumourigenesis

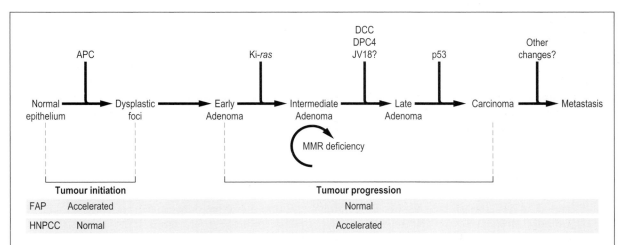

Fig. 13.15 Multi-step development of colonic cancer. The accumulation of as many as ten mutations in several tumour suppressor genes and oncogenes over a lifetime results in cancer. Adenoma, benign epithelial tumour; APC, adenomatous polyposis coli; Carcinoma, malignant epithelial tumour; DCC (deleted in colorectal cancer) DPC4, JV18 and p53, tumour suppressor gene products; dysplastic foci, regions of abnormal development; FAP, familial adematomatous polyposis; HNPCC, hereditary nonpolyposis colorectal cancer; Ki-*ras*, the Kirsten *ras* oncogene; MMR, mismatch repair gene products. Inactivating genetic events in each allele of the tumour suppressor genes are required. A single genetic event in one Ki-*ras* allele is sufficient for its activation. Comparison of mutation rates in FAP and HNPCC illustrates that different pathways of tumour development and progression can lead to similar cancers (adapted from Kinzler K W, Vogelstein B 1996 Cell 87: 159–170.)

Oncogenes and proto-oncogenes

Oncogenes were discovered as virally encoded genes that resulted in the loss of host cell growth control when expressed in virus-invaded cells. The proteins encoded by oncogenes are related to the products of non-oncogenic cellular genes, termed **proto-oncogenes**. The presence of oncogenes in viral genomes is thought to have occurred by recombination of ancestral viral genome with proto-oncogenes in the host cell followed by subsequent mutation into an active oncogene. Expression of cellular oncogenes or the abnormal expression of proto-oncogenes is thought to over-ride normal cell cycle control and lead to uncontrolled cell proliferation. This is clearly an advantage for the virus, which makes use of the host cell machinery for its replication.

Oncogenes may arise in cells due to:

- viral infection and the induction of increased virally encoded proto-oncogene expression under the control of the constitutively active viral promoter
- viral infection and expression of a virally encoded oncogene activated by mutation
- chromosomal translocation of cellular proto-oncogenes which place the gene under different transcriptional control, e.g. Burkitt's lymphoma and chronic myelogenous leukaemia (see box)
- mutation within the coding region of a cellular proto-oncogene, e.g. *ras* and *src* oncogenes (see box)
- loss of an inhibition of transformation, i.e. loss of an **anti-oncogene** or **tumour suppressor gene** activity, e.g. retinoblastoma susceptibility gene product (see below) and p53 (see box).

Most proto-oncogenes encode components of cellular signalling pathways. Their oncogenic potential arises from their ability to mimic growth factors, hormone receptors, G-proteins, intracellular signalling effector enzymes and transcription factors (Fig. 13.16), all of which ultimately lead to a modified control of key regulatory genes. It is noteworthy, for example, that over 30% of all human oncogenes encode tyrosine kinases which normally couple growth factor activation to cell proliferation.

Tumour suppressor genes

Tumour suppressor genes represent an additional and important family of proto-oncogenes. In normal cells their activity is anti-oncogenic, such that a loss of activity results in constitutive activation of cell growth. These genes encode proteins of unrelated functions which are normally involved in the regulation of normal cell division and differentiation (Table 13.2).

> #### Retinoblastoma
>
> The retinoblastoma susceptibility gene (*Rb*) is an example of a tumour suppressor gene, mutation of which results in retinal tumours in the young. Both copies of the *Rb* gene must be mutated for retinoblastoma to develop. In the more common inherited form the patient inherits one defective and one wild-type *Rb* allele. Mutation in the wild-type allele, due to the high mutation rate in this gene, results in two defective alleles and usually the development of bilateral retinoblastoma at a young age. Where there is no family history, a unilateral retinoblastoma may develop if both copies of the *Rb* gene become mutated in the same cell. The *Rb* gene product, pRb, is thought to control the passage of the cell from G_1 to S phase by binding E2F transcription factors (see Fig. 13.2). The deletion of pRb in retinoblastoma presumably leads to unchecked passage at the G_1–S phase checkpoint and, therefore, loss of control of the cell cycle. Interestingly, early tumours do not develop in other tissues in children with inherited retinoblastoma even when cells are homozygous for mutated pRb. Other factors are required for cancer to develop in these tissues. It is noteworthy that many incidences of inheritable retinoblastoma arise from *de novo* mutations in the germ line, rather than inheritance of an established defective allele.

Proto-oncogenes in normal cells

It must be remembered that potentially oncogenic genes, i.e. proto-oncogenes, have important functions in normal cells either in signalling and/or the regulation of cell differentiation.

Some oncogenes linked with human cancers

- In Burkitt's lymphoma the *c-myc* gene is translocated from chromosome 8 to chromosome 14, which places the proto-oncogene under the control of an active immunoglobulin locus.

- In patients with chronic myelogenous leukaemia the *c-abl* proto-oncogene is translocated from chromosome 8 to chromosome 22. In most patients this results in a novel fusion protein with a constitutively active tyrosine kinase activity.

- A single base change, leading to a single amino acid substitution, in the *ras* proto-oncogene results in transformation of the *ras* gene product into an oncogenic form. Different point mutations transform the *ras* proto-oncogene by different mechanisms, i.e. either by inhibiting endogenous GTP hydrolytic activity or by altering the rate of guanine nucleotide exchange.

- Deletion of part of the EGF receptor gene produces the *src* oncogene.

- Inactivation of the tumour suppressor gene product p53 is implicated in 50–60% of all human cancers. A wide range of mutations are found in p53 and different mutations are associated not only with different chemical inducers of cancer or radiation but also with different types of cancer.

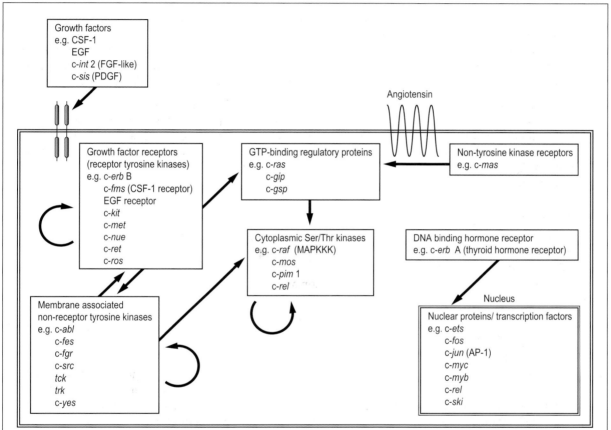

Fig. 13.16 Inter-relationships between proto-oncogenes involved in signalling pathways. Curly arrows indicate self-activation by autophosphorylation. CSF, colony stimulating factor; EGF, epidermal growth factor; FGF, fibroblast growth factor; PDGF, platelet-derived growth factor.

Gene product	Normal cell function	Oncogenic potential
pRb	Inhibition of E2F transcription factors	Unchecked passage bewteen G_1 and S phase resulting in transformation
CKI	Restrict activation of CDK and cell cycle	Unchecked activation of CDK
GAP	Increases the rate of GTP hydrolysis in *ras*, thereby reducing signal duration	Reduced rate of GTP hydrolysis by *ras* gene product leading to extended activation and mitogenic signalling
p53	Transcription factor expressed in response to DNA damage to check the cell cycle in G_1	Progression of cells containing damaged DNA through the cell cycle
Phosphotyrosine phosphatases	Reduction of mitogenic signals	Increased mitogenic tyrosine phosphorylation
TGFβ receptor	Anti-mitogenic signalling in response to TGFβ	Removal of tumour suppression
Transcription factors	Negative regulation of gene expression	Uncontrolled gene expression

Table 13.2 Some candidate anti-oncogenic or tumour suppressor genes. CDK, cyclin-dependent protein kinase; CKI, cyclin-dependent protein kinase inhibitors; GAP, GTPase activating proteins; p53, p53 tumour suppressor gene product

Apoptosis

Two types of cell death can be distinguished (Fig. 13.17). 'Accidental' cell death or **necrosis** occurs after severe and sudden injury. It is characterized by the swelling of organelles and a breakdown of the integrity of the plasma membrane, which results in the leakage of cellular contents and an inflammatory response. Programmed cell death or **apoptosis** occurs in response to physiological triggers in development (tissue remodelling), defence, homeostasis and ageing. Apoptotic cells initially shrink and lose microvilli and cell junctions. Organelles maintain their structure but the plasma membrane becomes highly convoluted and the cell breaks down into small apoptotic bodies, which are quickly phagocytosed by macrophages. This occurs without leakage of cellular constituents and, hence, without an inflammatory response. Apoptosis is often accompanied by a characteristic condensation and fragmentation of chromatin by endogenous endonuclease activity between centrosomes. This results in multiple DNA fragments, which appear as a ladder differing by 180–200 base pairs when analysed by electrophoresis.

Apoptosis in disease processes

Apoptosis may play important roles in many disease processes. An apoptotic response to DNA damage may protect tissues from viral infection. Apoptosis may be important in eliminating cells containing damaged DNA that may contribute to the initial development of cancer and in suppressing the neoplastic signals in others. Failure of apoptosis in these situations could contribute to the initiation of the tumourigenic process and the appearance of tumour cells resistant to cytotoxic therapy. Inappropriate induction of apoptosis may contribute significantly to degenerative diseases, and failure to deplete self-reactive T cells by apoptosis may be important in the development of autoimmune disease.

Mechanisms of programmed cell death

Mechanisms signalling apoptosis in cells remain to be elucidated but are clearly very varied (Fig. 13.18). Signals for apoptosis in one cell type can induce cell proliferation and differentiation in other cell types. Raised $[Ca^{2+}]_i$ and increased mRNA and protein synthesis, including that of cell cycle regulatory genes, proto-oncogenes (e.g. c-*myc*, c-*fos* and c-*jun*) and tumour suppressors (e.g. p53), are commonly but not universally implicated in apoptosis. Whether implicated gene products induce cell proliferation or apoptosis probably depends on their associations with other proteins and reflects the complexity and fine balance of the regulation of the cell cycle.

Important molecular candidates implicated in the apoptotic process include:

- p53. One role of apoptosis may be to remove cells containing irreversibly damaged DNA. DNA damage induces the production of p53, a transcription factor that results in the arrest of the cell cycle in G_1 to allow DNA repair. Should repair fail, p53 may trigger cell removal by apoptosis.
- Interleukin-1β-converting enzymes (ICE). Proteoloysis of cell constituents is characteristic of apoptosis and overexpression of ICE cysteine proteases has been demonstrated to induce apoptotic cell death.
- Bcl-2. This protein suppresses some apoptotic pathways and a reduction in Bcl-2 levels has been associated with apoptosis.

Cell senescence

Cell senescence or ageing may be associated with repetitive DNA sequences, **telomeres**, that are found at the ends of chromosomes. Telomeres are not replicated in the same way as the body of chromosomal DNA but are synthesized by the enzyme **telomerase**, which is less exacting and produces random variation in the number of repeats of telomeric DNA sequence. Cell senescence is associated with a shortening of telomeres, possibly due to the absence of telomerase in somatic cells. This process limits the maximum number of cell divisions of any cell, but why cells should age in this way is not known.

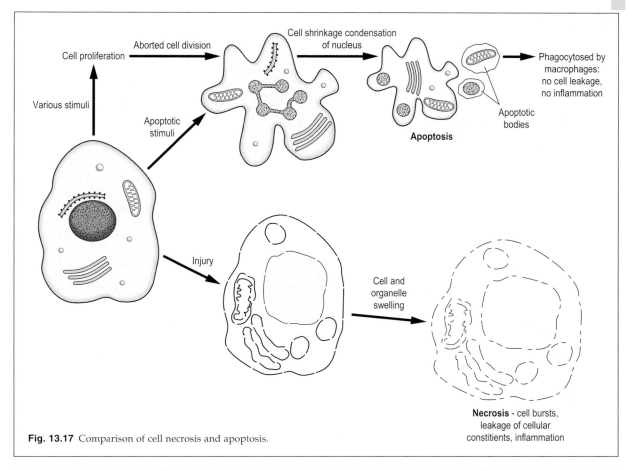

Fig. 13.17 Comparison of cell necrosis and apoptosis.

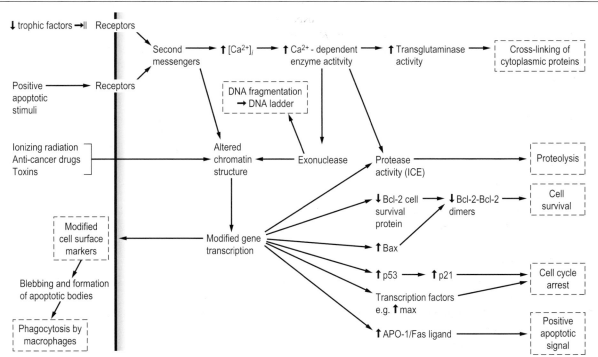

Fig. 13.18 A model for the integration of signals leading to apoptosis. Characteristic apoptotic end points are shown in bold type. Positive apoptotic stimuli include APO-1/Fas ligand, glucocorticoids, human immunodeficiency virus protein gp120, transforming growth factor β (TGF-β) and tumour necrosis factor (TNF). Note: apoptotic signals are not universal for all cell types, indeed the same signalling molecule may stimulate cell proliferation in other cells. Bax, a protein related to Bcl-2, can interact with Bcl-2 and thereby accelerate apoptosis. The Bcl-2/Bax ratio may contribute to the control of whether a cell becomes apoptotic. p21 is a cyclin-dependent protein kinase inhibitor. ICE, interleukin-1β-converting enzyme.

Further reading

Edwards R G, Brody S A 1995 Principles and practice of assisted human reproduction. W B Saunders, Philadelphia

Grana X, Reddy E P 1995 Cell cycle control in mammalian cells: role of cyclins, cyclin-dependent kinases (CDKs), growth suppressor genes and cyclin-dependent kinase inhibitors (CKIs). Oncogene 11: 211–219

Hale A J, Smith C A, Sutherland L C et al 1996 Apoptosis: molecular regulation of cell death. European Journal of Biochemistry 236: 1–26

Majano G, Joris I 1995 Apoptosis, oncosis, and necrosis: an overview of cell death. Americal Journal of Pathology 146: 3–15

Mendelsohn J, Howley P M, Israel M A, Liotta L A 1995 The molecular basis of cancer. W B Saunders, Philadelphia.

Morgan D O 1995 Principles of CDK regulation. Nature 374: 131–133

Murray A, Hunt T 1993 The cell cycle: an introduction. Oxford University Press, New York

Orrenius S 1995 Apoptosis: molecular mechanisms and implications for human disease. Journal of Internal Medicine 237: 529–536

Snell W J, White J M 1996 The molecules of mammalian fertilization. Cell 85: 629–637

Stillman B 1996 Cell-cycle control of DNA-replication. Science 274: 1659–1664

Thompson C B 1995 Apoptosis in the pathogenesis and treatment of disease. Science 267: 1456–1462

Revision questions

1. Outline the phases of the cell cycle indicating the main events of each stage. At what point may cells become quiescent and cease to divide?

2. On a diagram of the cell cycle indicate where cyclin-dependent protein kinases are important for the passage between stages.

3. Outline the similarities and differences in the replication of DNA on the leading (5′ to 3′) and lagging (3′ to 5′) strands of double-helical DNA.

4. Why is cell cycle arrest important?

5. Outline the mechanisms of DNA repair in cells.

6. In a mitotic cell, describe the major anatomical changes that are apparent in interphase, prophase, prometaphase metaphase, anaphase, telophase and cytokinesis.

7. How do the first and second meiotic divisions differ?

8. In oogenesis how many viable oocytes result from meiotic division from a progenitor cell?

9. Outline the important features of fertilization.

10. What is the difference between an oncogene and a proto-oncogene? In what ways do oncogenes lead to tumourigenesis?

11. Why do cells become cancerous?

12. What is apoptosis? How does apoptosis contribute to tissue physiology? How can cells undergoing apoptosis be distinguished from necrotic cells?

Answers to revision questions

1. The cell cycle comprises a period of preparation for nuclear division (interphase) and a period of nuclear and cell division (M phase). Interphase, the period between cell divisions, can be further subdivided into G_1 phase, S phase and G_2 phase. G_1 phase is a period of rapid biosynthesis and growth to provide the constituents for a new cell. During S phase the complete genome is duplicated. The cell is then prepared for cell division during G_2 phase, after which it enters M phase where the nuclear material is divided (mitosis) and cytoplasmic division (cytokinesis) into two new cells occurs. Cells may become quiescent after M phase when they are said to be in G_0 phase.

2. See Fig. 13.2.

3. After the double-helical structure is unwound, DNA synthesis against both DNA strands requires the synthesis of short complementary RNA primers by RNA polymerases. DNA polymerase III then catalyses the synthesis of a complementary DNA strand against the template DNA strands in the 5'–3' direction. As more DNA unwinds, synthesis against the leading strand can continue uninterrupted. Synthesis against the newly exposed lagging strand, however, requires synthesis of further RNA primers such that a series of discontinuous DNA fragments (Okazaki fragments) are made. To complete the sister DNA strand against the lagging strand the RNA primers are removed by RNase H and the DNA strand is completed by DNA polymerase I. The fragments are then joined by DNA ligase to produce the final sister DNA molecule.

4. Cell cycle arrest is important to provide a safeguard to prevent genetically damaged cells from being reproduced.

5. Simple lesions, such as the alkylation of bases, can be reversed simply by enzyme catalysed repair. Other lesions are repaired by excision repair where the removal of the damaged base or a short stretch of sequence containing the damaged base(s) is followed by the replacement of new sequence against the template of the undamaged strand.

6. In interphase each chromosome is duplicated. In prophase the joined sister chromatids condense, the nucleolus is disassembled and the mitotic spindle begins to form on the nuclear envelope from cytoskeletal elements. In prometaphase the nuclear membrane fragments and the chromosomes associate with the growing mitotic spindle and begin to orientate on the spindle at right angles. Metaphase is when all the chromosomes are aligned at the centre of the mitotic spindle. In anaphase the centromeres split into two and the paired chromosomes migrate to opposite poles of the mitotic spindle. Telophase is the end of mitosis where the nuclear membrane and nucleoli reform. Cytokinesis starts in late anaphase by the formation of a cleavage furrow of actomyosin, which deepens progressively until the opposing edges of the cell meet and membrane fusion results in the generation of two new cells.

7. Before the first meiotic division the chromatin of the progenitor cell is duplicated and the sister chromatids remain joined at the centrosome. During this division, homologous chromosomes pair and recombination events occur between the pairs, resulting in some mixing of genetic material from the two parental chromosomes. At division, the pairs of chromosomes separate (the sister chromatids remain associated). During the second meiotic division there is no DNA replication and sister chromatids separate at their centromeres.

8. A single viable haploid oocyte and three non-viable polar bodies are produced. During both meiotic divisions the cytoplasmic constituents are divided asymmetrically producing a well-nourished cell and a polar body. Polar bodies from the first meiotic division divide into two further polar bodies in the second meiotic division.

9. Recognition of the zona pellucida of the oocyte triggers a large influx of Ca^{2+} into the bound sperm, which induces the release of hydrolytic enzymes. These digest the zona pellucida allowing the sperm to penetrate to the plasma membrane by virtue of the extension of an acrosomal process. When sperm and oocyte membranes meet, they fuse. Fusion stimulates the release of oocyte cortical granules containing enzymes that modify the zona pellucida, rendering it impenetrable to further sperm. The sperm nucleus is transferred and a rise in $[Ca^{2+}]_i$ in the fertilized oocyte triggers the progression of meiosis from metaphase II.

10. An oncogene is a gene that, in combination with other oncogenes, can result in the transformation of a normal cell into a tumourigenic cell. A proto-oncogene is a gene that has the potential, if mutated, to become an oncogene.

11. Cells become cancerous as a result of loss of growth control due to the activation of oncogenes. Cellular oncogenes arise by mutation of proto-oncogenes in somatic cells. It is also possible that some human cancers arise as a result of infection by viruses containing oncogenes in their genome. A cell must accumulate several oncogenic mutations before full transformation into a cancerous cell occurs. Oncogenes lead to uncontrolled cell growth either by providing a constant mitogenic signal or by removing normal mechanisms that prevent uncontrolled entry into the cell cycle.

12. Apoptosis is programmed cell death and occurs in response to physiological stimuli, rather than cell injury. Apoptosis contributes to processes of tissue remodelling, such as in tissue development, defence mechanisms, tissue homeostasis and ageing, by removing unwanted cells. Apoptotic cells shrink and lose microvilli and cell junctions and their chromatin is often condensed and fragmented. Organelles remain intact but the plasma membrane becomes highly convoluted and small apoptotic bodies break off. This occurs without cell leakage. Necrotic cells, by comparison, have swollen organelles and become leaky as a result of a breakdown in the integrity of the plasma membrane.

Abbreviations

A band anisotropic band
ABC ATP-binding cassette
AC adenylyl cyclase
ACh acetylcholine
AChR acetylcholine receptor
ACTH adrenocorticotrophic hormone
ADP adenosine 5′ diphosphate
AKAP A-kinase anchoring protein
AMP adenosine 5′ monophosphate
AMPA α-amino-3-hydroxy-5-methyl-4-isoxazoleproprionate
ANP atrial natriuretic peptide
APC adenomatous polyposis coli
AP sites DNA nucleotide sites lacking bases
ARF Monomeric G-protein associated with vesicle transport
ATP adenosine 5′ triphosphate
ATPase adenosine 5′ triphosphatase
βARK β-adrenoceptor protein kinase
BP billous pemphigoid protein (blistering disease autoantigens)
BSE bovine spongioform encephalopathy
[Ca^{2+}]$_i$ intracellular free calcium concentration
CAM cellular adhesion molecule
CAM-kinase Ca^{2+}-calmodulin-dependent protein kinase
cA-PK cyclic AMP-dependent protein kinase
Ca^{2+} pump plasma membrane Ca^{2+}–Mg^{2+}-ATPase
CD45 leucocyte common antigen
CDK cyclin-dependent protein kinase
cDNA complementary (copy) deoxyribonucleic acid
CFTR cystic fibrosis transmembrane conductance regulator
cG-PK cyclic GMP-dependent protein kinase
CKI cyclin-dependent protein kinase inhibitor
CLC anion (Cl$^-$) selective channels
CLIP corticotrophin-like intermediate lobe peptide
CNS central nervous system
COX-1 cyclo-oxygenase 1
COX-2 cyclo-oxygenase 2
CSF colony stimulating factor
CTK cytoplasmic tyrosine kinase
CURL compartment for the uncoupling of receptor and ligand
cyclic AMP cyclic adenosine 3′,5′ monophosphate
cyclic GMP cyclic guanosine 3′,5′ monophosphate
DAG 1,2-diacylglycerol
DCC deleted in colorectal cancer
ddATP dideoxy-ATP
ddNTP dideoxy-nucleotide triphosphate
DMD Duchenne muscular dystrophy

DNA deoxyribonucleic acid
E$_{Ca}$ calcium equilibrium potential
ECM extracellular matrix
E. coli *Escherichia coli*
EDRF endothelium-derived relaxing factor
EF-1 elongation factor-1
EF-Tu elongation factor-Tu
EGF epidermal growth factor
E$_K$ potassium equilibrium potential
ELISA enzyme-linked immunosorbent assay
E$_{Na}$ sodium equilibrium potential
EPSP excitatory postsynaptic potential
ER endoplasmic reticulum
FACS fluorescence activated cell sorting
F-actin actin filament polymers
FAD (FAD2H) flavin adenine dinucleotide (reduced form)
FAP familial adenatomatous polyposis
GABA gamma amino butyric acid
G-actin monomeric actin
GAG glycosaminoglycan
Gal galactose
GAP GTPase activating proteins
GDP guanosine diphosphate
G$_g$ G-protein in taste buds
G$_i$ inhibitory G-protein (for adenylyl cyclase)
Glc glucose
GlcNac N-acetyl-glucosamine
GLP-1 glucagon-like peptide 1
GLUT glucose transporter
Gly glycine
G-1-P glucose-1-phosphate
G-6-P glucose-6-phosphate
G$_L$ liver glycogen targeting proteins
G$_M$ muscle glycogen targeting proteins
GMP guanosine monophosphate
GNRP guanine-nucleotide releasing protein
G$_0$ G-protein in brain, couples to Ca^{2+} channels
G$_{olf}$ G-protein coupled to odourant receptors
gp glycoprotein
GP glycogen phosphorylase
G-protein GTP-binding regulatory protein
G$_q$ G-proteins coupled to phospholipase C
Grb2 SH2 and SH3 domain containing signal transducing protein
GRK G-protein receptor protein kinase
G$_s$ stimulatory G-protein (for adenylyl cyclase)
GS glycogen synthetase
G$_t$ transducin
GTP guanosine triphosphate
GTPase guanosine triphosphatase
H-bonds hydrogen bonds
HLH helix–loop–helix
HNPCC hereditary non-polyposis colorectal cancer

H₂O₂	hydrogen peroxide
HPETE	hydroperoxyeicosatetraenoic acid
5-HT	5-hydroxytryptamine
HYPP	hyperkalaemic periodic paralysis
I band	isotropic band
ICAM	inter-cellular adhesion molecule
ICE	interleukin-1β-converting enzyme
ICSI	intracytoplasmic sperm injection
Ig	immunoglobulin
IgA	immunoglobulin A
IGF	insulin-like growth factor
InsP₃	inositol 1,4,5-trisphosphate
InsP₄	inositol 1,3,4,5-tetrakisphosphate
IPSP	inhibitory postsynaptic potential
IRS-1	insulin receptor substrate-1
ISPK	insulin-sensitive protein kinase
K_D	dissociation constant
K_DR	delayed rectifier K⁺ channel
K_IR	inward rectifier K⁺ channel
Ki-ras	Kirsten *ras* oncogene
K_M	Michaelis constant
LAR	leucocyte common antigen related protein
LDL	low density lipoprotein
LHON	Leber's hereditary optic neuropathy
LTB₄	leukotriene B₄
LTC₄	leukotriene C₄
LTD₄	leukotriene D₄
LTE₄	leukotriene E₄
β-LPH	β-lipotrophin
γ-LPH	γ-lipotrophin
mAChR	muscarinic acetylcholine receptor
MAP-1C	cytoplasmic dynein
MAP-2	microtubule-associated protein 2
MAPs	microtubule-associated proteins
MAPK	mitogen-activated protein kinase
MAPKK	mitogen-activated protein kinase kinase
MAPKKK	mitogen-activated protein kinase kinase kinase
MDR1	multidrug resistance protein 1
MEK	mitogen-activated protein kinase kinase kinase
MELAS	myoclonus encephalopathy with stroke-like episodes
MEPP	miniature endplate potential
MERRF	myoclonus, epilepsy with ragged fibres
MLC	myosin light chain
MLCK	myosin light chain kinase
MMP	matrix metalloproteinase
MMR	mismatch repair gene products
MPF	mitosis-promoting factor
mRNA	messenger ribonucleic acid
MSD	membrane spanning domain
α-MSH	α-melanocyte-stimulating hormone
MTOC	microtubule organizing centre
Na⁺ pump	Na⁺-K⁺-ATPase
nAChR	nicotinic acetylcholine receptor
NAD⁺ (NADH)	nicotinamide adenine dinucleotide (reduced form)

NANA	N-acyl neuraminic acid (sialic acid)
NCAM	neural cell adhesion molecule
NF	neurofilament
NHE	Na⁺–H⁺ exchange
NMDA	N-methyl-D-aspartate
NO	nitric oxide
NOS	nitric oxide synthase
NSAID	non-steroidal anti-inflammatory drug
NSF protein	N-ethylmaleimide-sensitive fusion protein
p	protein
p53a	tumour suppressor gene product
PAM	potassium-aggravated myotonia
PC	paramyotonia congenita
PCR	polymerase chain reaction
PDGF	platelet-derived growth factor
PDI	protein disulphide isomerase
PGD₂	prostaglandin D₂
PGE₂	prostaglandin E₂
PGI₂	prostaglandin I₂
PhK	phosphorylase kinase
P_i	inorganic phosphate
PKA	cyclic AMP-dependent protein kinase
PKC	protein kinase C
PLC	phospholipase C
PLD	phospholipase D
PMCA	plasma membrane Ca²⁺–Mg²⁺-ATPase
P_o	open probability
POMC	pro-opiomelanocorticotrophin
PPase	protein phosphatases
pRb	retinoblastoma tumour suppressor gene product
PP1G	G subunit of protein phosphatase-1
PtdCho	phosphatidylcholine
PtdIns	phosphatidylinositol
PtdInsP	phosphatidylinositol 4-phosphate
PtdInsP₂	phosphatidylinositol 4,5-bisphosphate
Rab	monomeric G-protein associated with vesicle transport
Ran1	monomeric G-protein associated with nuclear protein import
Ras	monomeric G-protein
RFLP	restriction fragment length polymorphism
Rho	monomeric G-protein associated with cytoskeletons
RIA	radioimmunoassay
RNA	ribonucleic acid
RNase	ribonuclease
ROC	receptor-operated channel
RTK	receptor tyrosine kinase
RT-PCR	reverse transcriptase polymerase chain reaction
RyR	ryanodine receptor
SDS	sodium dodecyl sulphate
SDS-PAGE	SDS-polyacrylamide gel electrophoresis
SERCA	sarco(endo)plasmic reticulum Ca²⁺-ATPase

sGC   soluble guanylyl cyclase
SH2 domain   *src* homology 2 domain
SH3 domain   *src* homology 3 domain
sLe   sialyl Lewis
SLRPs   small leucine-rich proteoglycans
SNAP   N-ethylmaleimide sensitive fusion attachment protein
SNARE   SNAP receptor
Sos   signal transducing protein
SR   sarcoplasmic reticulum
SRP   signal recognition particle
SSR   signal sequence receptor
SUR   sulphonylurea receptor
T$_3$ and T$_4$ thyroid hormones
TATA box   eukaryotic promoter sequence
TEA$^+$ triethylammonium ion
TGFβ   transforming growth factor β
TIMPs   tissue inhibitors of metalloproteinases
7TMDR   seven transmembrane domain receptors

TnC   Ca^{2+}-binding subunit of troponin
TNF   tumour necrosis factor
TnL   actin-binding subunit of troponin
TnT   tropomyosin-binding subunit of troponin
tRNA   transfer ribonucleic acid
tSNARE   target membrane SNAP receptor
dTTP   deoxythymidine triphosphate
t-tubule   transverse tubule
TXA$_2$ thromboxane A$_2$
UDP   uridine diphosphate
UTR   untranslated region
UV   ultraviolet
VAMP   synaptobrevin
VASP   vasodilator-stimulated phosphoprotein
VCAM   vascular cell adhesion molecule
V$_m$ membrane potential
V$_{max}$ maximum initial rate
vSNARE   vesicle SNAP receptor
Wee1   cyclin-dependent protein kinase

Tools of molecular cell biology: biochemical, cell biological and immunological

Microscopy

Cells and larger cellular components may either absorb or deflect incident waveforms allowing them to be 'visualized'. Visualization may be made directly using light microscopy or indirectly by electron microscopy (Table A2.1).

	Light microscopy	Electron microscopy
Wavelength of incident radiation	400–700 nm	0.004 nm
Magnification	Up to 2000 times	Up to 400 000 times
Resolution	> 0.2 μm	> 1–2 nm
	Cellular morphology and some subcellular structures	Subcellular structures and some macromolecules
Tissues	Living or dead tissue	Dead/fixed tissues only
Modes of operation	Unstained (phase contrast) or stained (bright field) preparations	Requires staining or low-angle shadowing with electron-dense stains to 'visualize' structures

Table A2.1 Comparison of light and electron microscopy

Tissue and cell culture

Experimentally it is often advantageous to simplify the experimental system from the whole organism to an isolated tissue or single cell type. This is achieved by growing tissue biopsies or dissociated cells in vitro in sterile nutrient medium containing growth factors to maintain cell viability. When required growth factors are present in the medium, cells will continue to divide and, in principle, the production of large numbers of cells is possible. For cell culture, individual cells are dissociated from tissues using proteolytic enzyme treatments, usually **chymotrypsin**. Individual cells round-up after dissociation but quickly settle and adhere to the plastic substratum of the culture dish. In so doing, cells generally flatten and take on a more physiological morphology. Animal cells in culture will continue to divide until a confluent monolayer is formed in the dish, when **contact inhibition** represses further cell division. In **transformed** or cancerous cells this contact inhibition is lost and cells overgrow each other. Cells may continue to maintain their differentiated structures and functions through many cell divisions or **passages**. With increasing passage number, however, there is an increased risk of de-differentiation to a fibroblastic form. This is an important consideration when studying a function of differentiated cells.

Fluorescence activated cell sorting (FACS)

Individual cells may be sorted on the basis of antigens that they present on their cell surface. Cell antigens are first labelled with antibodies coupled to a fluorescent dye. Labelled cells are streamed dropwise through a fluorescence detector such that each drop contains only a single cell. Depending on whether or not fluorescence is detected, droplets are given either a positive or negative charge by the sorter. Further passage of the cells through a strong electric field then deflects cells into collection tubes depending on the charge on the droplet.

Subcellular fractionation (Fig. A2.1)

Cells are disrupted usually by applying shear forces in a homogenizer. Use of an isotonic buffer protects organelles from substantial lysis. Subcellular fractions are collected by sequential centrifugation steps using increasing angular momentum and run times to sediment organelles of progressively lower buoyant density. Alternatively, by using a continuous density gradient (e.g. of sucrose of Percoll) in the centrifuge tube, subcellular fractions of different buoyant densities may be separated by their banding position in the gradient after centrifugation.

Protein separation

Proteins may be separated from each other by **column chromatography** (Fig. A2.2) and **electrophoresis** (Fig. A2.3).

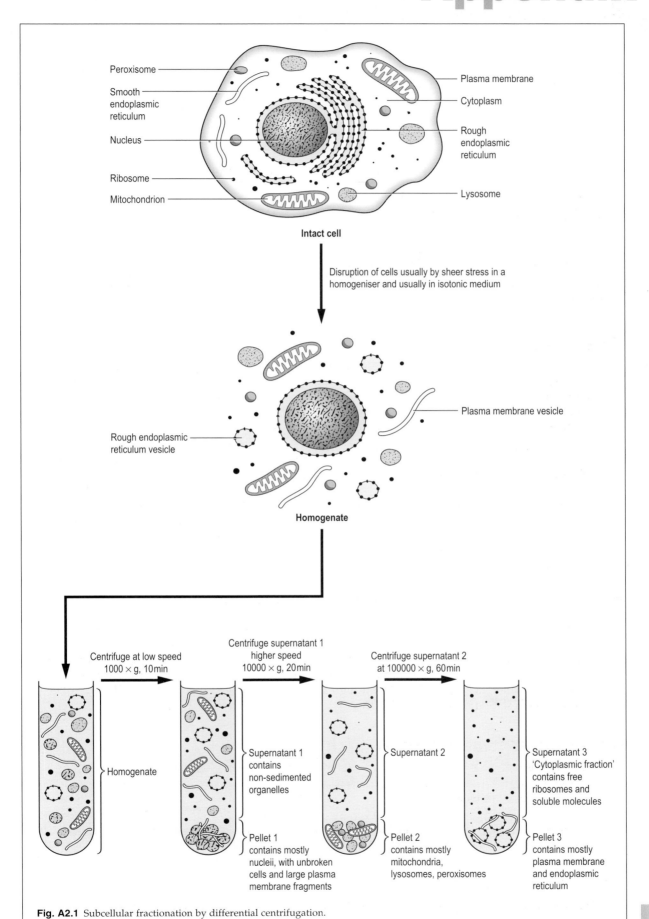

Fig. A2.1 Subcellular fractionation by differential centrifugation.

Appendix 2

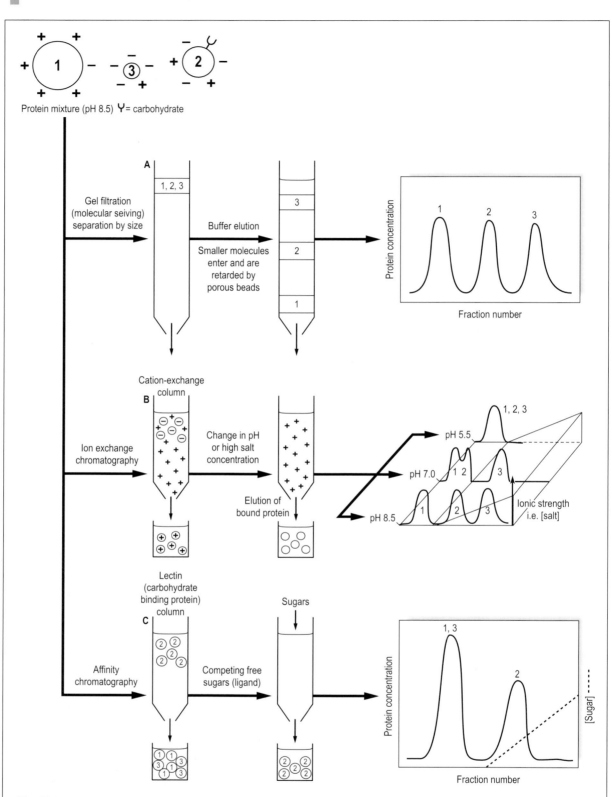

Fig. A2.2 Separation and purification of proteins. Proteins may be separated on the basis of **size**, by gel filtration (panel a) or gradient centrifugation, **charge**, by ion-exchange chromatography (panel b), isoelectric focusing and electrophoresis (see Fig A2.3) or **specific properties**, e.g. affinity chromatography based on ligand binding, attached carbohydrate moieties (panel c) or epitopes for immune recognition (see Fig. A2.6e–g). (a) During gel filtration, smaller proteins enter the porous beads while larger proteins are excluded. Small proteins are retarded by the beads while excluded proteins pass round the beads and elute more quickly. (b) In ion-exchange chromatography, charged beads form ionic bonds with proteins of opposite charge, thereby retarding their elution. Bound proteins may be eluted by an increase in salt concentration, to compete with ionic interactions, or a change in pH, which may change the charge on bound proteins due to the association or dissociation of H$^+$ ions from titratable groups (amino and carboxylic acid groups). (c) Specific binding of protein to ligand covalently attached to chromatography beads forms the basis of affinity chromatography. Bound proteins may be eluted in the presence of an excess of free ligand.

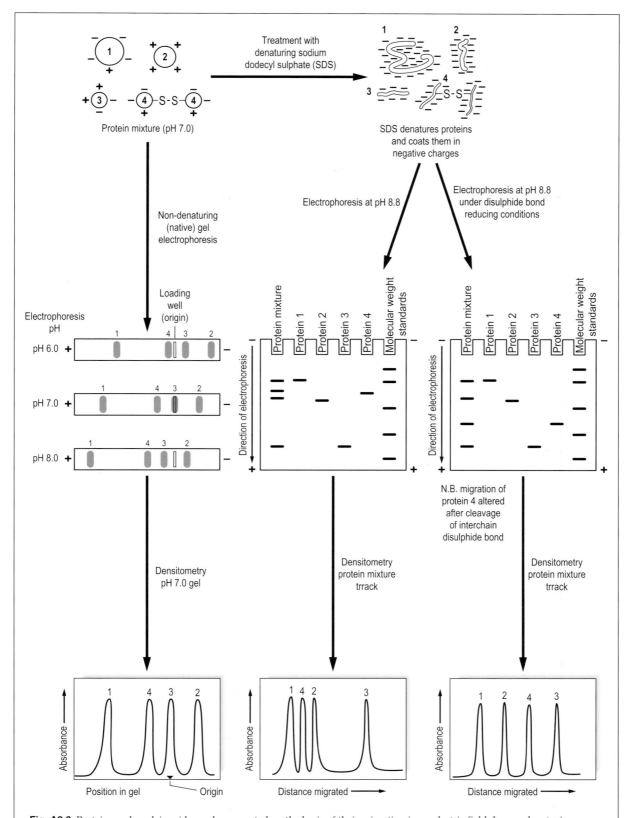

Fig. A2.3 Proteins and nucleic acids can be separated on the basis of their migration in an electric field. In non-denaturing (native) gel electrophoresis proteins migrate towards the anode or cathode depending on the charge on the protein at the operating pH. Note: by changing the pH the migration of proteins in native gel electrophoresis can be modified; the more acid the pH, the more positively charged the protein. The size and shape of the protein also influences its migration through the gel. Treatment with sodium dodecyl sulphate (SDS) denatures proteins and coats them with negative charges. Electrophoresis in SDS-polyacrylamide gels (SDS-PAGE) results in all proteins migrating towards the cathode and a separation by the gel matrix on the basis of size; smaller proteins migrate further. Treatment of proteins with reducing agents prior to SDS-PAGE cleaves disulphide bonds.

Immunological methods

The preparation of polyclonal and monoclonal antibodies is shown in Fig. A2.4. Injection of an animal, usually mice or rabbits, with a suspension of foreign protein results in the generation of an immune response against the protein. Serum taken from the animal will contain a mixture of antibodies directed against different epitopes on the protein, each produced by a different clone of B lymphocytes i.e. **polyclonal antibodies**. Alternatively, B lymphocytes from the spleen may be fused with rapidly dividing myeloma cells to produce immortalized hybridoma cells. Plating at high dilution in multiwell plates allows clones derived from single hybridoma cells to be isolated. The antibodies secreted from an individual monoclonal cell line are all directed against the same epitope and are termed **monoclonal antibodies**.

Antibody applications

Enzyme-linked immunosorbent assay (ELISA)

This permits antibody titre (activity) to be assessed (Fig. A2.5). In the simplest case, antigen is adsorbed in the wells of a 96-well plate and an 'antibody sandwich' is constructed by the sequential addition of primary antibody (directed against the antigen) and secondary antibody (directed against the primary antibody) conjugated to an enzyme detection system. Wells develop colour in proportion to the amount of bound primary antibody. Where two antibodies directed against different epitopes on the antigen are available, antibody 1 may be adsorbed into the well and antigen applied as part of the 'sandwich'.

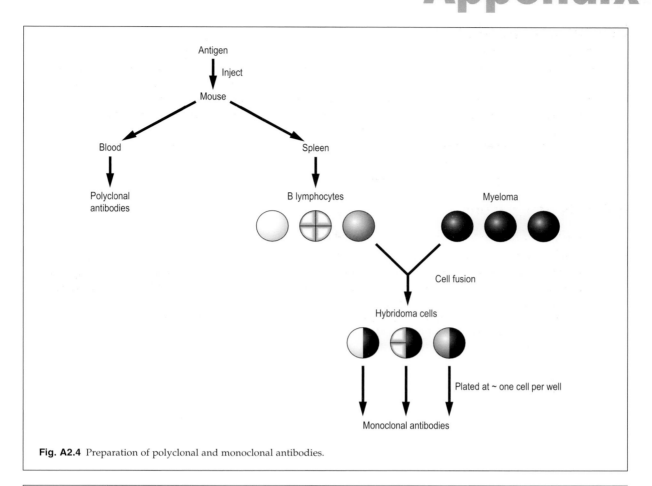

Fig. A2.4 Preparation of polyclonal and monoclonal antibodies.

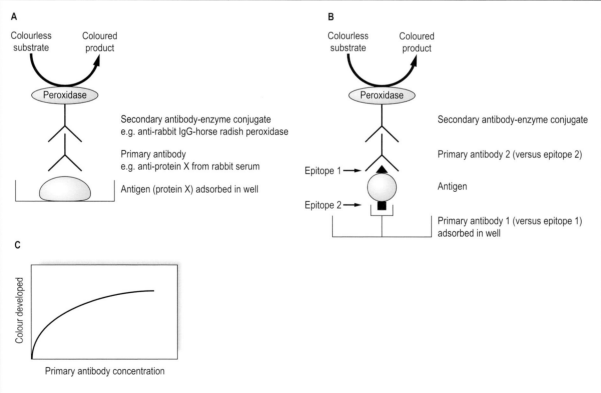

Fig. A2.5 Enzyme-linked immunosorbent assay (ELISA). A positive signal in any well is dependent on the binding of primary antibody to the antigen to permit the formation of the antibody sandwich detection system (**A–C**). In double antibody ELISA (**B**), the concentration of antigen determines the strength of the signal.

Appendix 2

Immunoprecipitation

Antibody–antigen complexes can be precipitated as crosslinked complexes, at the **equivalence point**, if approximately equimolar concentrations of antibody and antigen are used (Fig. A2.6B). Alternatively, addition of an excess of a secondary antibody against the primary antibody (Fig. A2.6D) or bead-immobilized primary (Fig. A2.6E) or secondary antibody (Fig. A2.6F) or antibody-binding protein A (Fig. A2.6G) can be used to effect immunoprecipitation.

Radioimmunoassay (RIA)

This permits the concentration of an unlabelled antigen in solution to be quantified by competition for binding to antibody with a fixed concentration of labelled antigen (Fig. A2.7). Antibody–antigen complexes are separated from free antigen by immunoprecipitation and the amount of immunoprecipitated label is quantified. The signal obtained in the presence of an unknown concentration of unlabelled antigen, e.g. from a patient, is calibrated by comparison with a standard curve of known concentrations of displacing antigen. RIA is often used for small polypeptides, e.g. hormones.

Western blotting or immunoblotting

This permits the identification of a specific polypeptide present in a mixture of proteins (Fig. A2.8). Proteins are separated electrophoretically and transferred to a 'filter'. Specific antibody recognition is used to localize staining or radioactivity (e.g. [^{125}I]protein A, an antibody-binding protein) to the band in the gel corresponding to the polypeptide of interest using an 'antibody sandwich'.

Immunocytochemistry

Antibody sandwich methods can be used as above to precipitate stain on localized antigen in tissue slices.

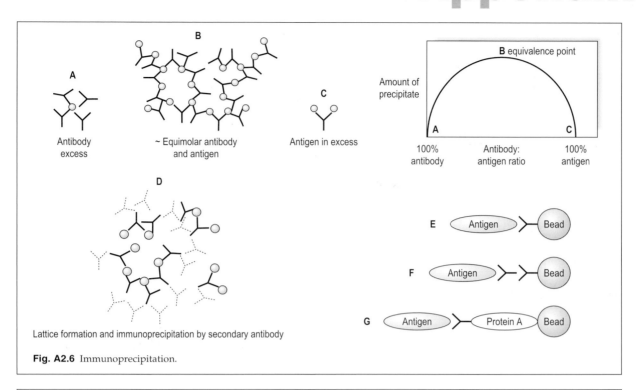

Fig. A2.6 Immunoprecipitation.

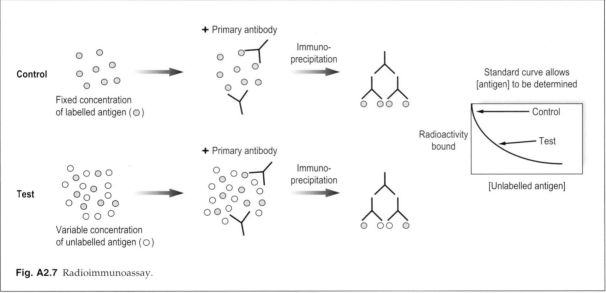

Fig. A2.7 Radioimmunoassay.

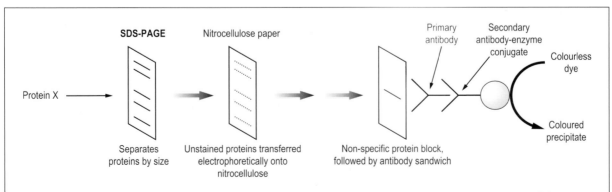

Fig. A2.8 Western blotting or immunoblotting. After transfer of electrophoretically separated proteins to the nitrocellulose paper, remaining protein adsorption sites are blocked with non-specific protein, such as casein, before application of the antibody detection system.

Tools of molecular cell biology: genetic methods

Gene cloning

In order to study the structure of a gene it is necessary to isolate it from other genes. The most common method of achieving this is to make a **gene library** and screen it for clones containing the gene of interest. Libraries can be made from the entire genome of the organism (genomic) (Fig. A3.1) or just from those genes that are expressed (transcribed) in a particular tissue at a particular time (cDNA). DNA molecules may be manipulated by using restriction endonucleases. These enzymes recognize specific sequences in the DNA molecule and cut it wherever they occur (Fig. A3.2). Fragments of DNA may be joined together by DNA ligase. Fragments of DNA may be ligated into either **plasmids** (autonomously replicating circular DNA molecules found in bacteria and yeast) or **bacteriophages** (viruses that infect bacteria) and propagated by transformation of *Escherichia coli*. The foreign DNA is faithfully replicated by the host bacteria and individual clones may be selected by colony hybridization with a suitable probe (see below). Plasmid or phage DNA containing the fragment of interest can be isolated from bacteria for sequencing or further manipulation.

DNA sequencing

The key to the function of a gene is its DNA sequence. This provides the derived primary sequence of the protein that it encodes and by comparison with other known sequences in a database may give clues to what the protein does. Analysis of the region immediately upstream (5′) of the transcription start site may also reveal how the gene is regulated.

Sequence analysis involves the synthesis of a new strand of DNA (complementary to the template strand) in the presence of a limiting concentration of **dideoxy-nucleotides** (ddNTPs). When one of these modified bases is incorporated into the growing DNA chain by the polymerase enzyme, its chemical structure blocks the addition of further nucleotides. If, for example, the reaction is carried out with a mixture of normal nucleotides plus a dideoxy-nucleotide, e.g. ddATP, then a series of chains of differing length will be produced, each one terminated where ddATP has been incorporated in place of dATP. If reactions are performed separately with each of the four ddNTPs and the newly synthesized DNA chains labelled radioactively, then the sequence of the template can be read by separating these DNA molecules on an acrylamide gel and visualizing the radioactivity with X-ray film (Fig. A3.3). This process has been simplified and automated by the introduction of ddNTPs that each carry a different fluorescent label. Now, all four bases can be used simultaneously in the same reaction and analysed on the same lane of a gel.

Southern blotting

Southern blotting (Fig. A3.4) takes advantage of the tendency of complementary strands of DNA or RNA to anneal together to form a double-stranded molecule. This process is referred to as **hybridization** and is dependent on both temperature and the concentration of monovalent cations, i.e. Na⁺. This process can occur with both strands in solution or with one immobilized on a nylon membrane.

Genomic or other DNA can be digested with restriction endonucleases to yield specific smaller fragments which may be separated according to their size by agarose gel electrophoresis. The fragments are then denatured to form single strands by treatment of the gel with alkali. After neutralization the fragments are transferred by capillary action to a special nylon membrane producing, in effect, a copy of the gel. Once the DNA has been fixed to the membrane (usually by crosslinking with ultraviolet light), the filter may be incubated with a single-stranded probe (DNA, RNA or an oligonucleotide, usually labelled with radioactivity). Where the sequence of the DNA on the filter is complementary to that of the probe then hybridization will occur. After the non-hybridizing probe has been removed by washing, hybridizing bands may be visualized on X-ray film by autoradiography.

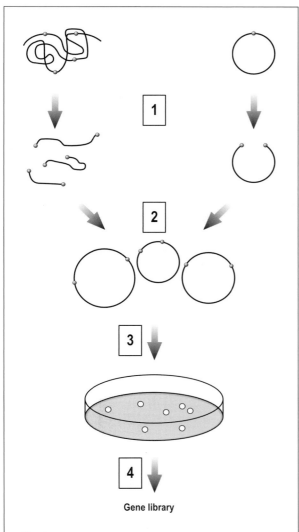

Fig. A3.1 Making a simple gene library. Step 1: Digestion of sample DNA and vector with a restriction endonuclease. Step 2: Ligation of sample DNA fragments into vector. Step 3: Transformation of *E. coli* and selection of transformants. Step 4: Propagation and analysis of recombinants.

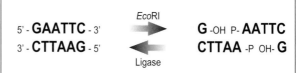

Fig. A3.2 Cutting and joining DNA molecules. Restriction endonucleases (such as *Eco*RI) recognise specific DNA sequences (normally short palindromic sequences i.e. they have the same sequence on each strand, e.g. GAATTC or GGATCC), cutting both DNA strands. DNA molecules can be joined together in a reaction catalysed by DNA ligase.

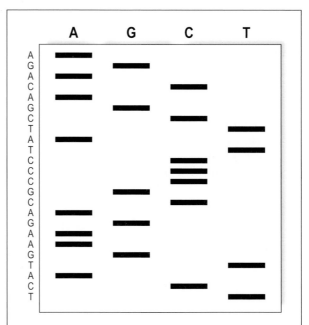

Fig. A3.3 A DNA sequencing gel. The sequence of the DNA template is read from the ladder of bands (starting at the bottom of the gel – T,C,A,T,G,A...).

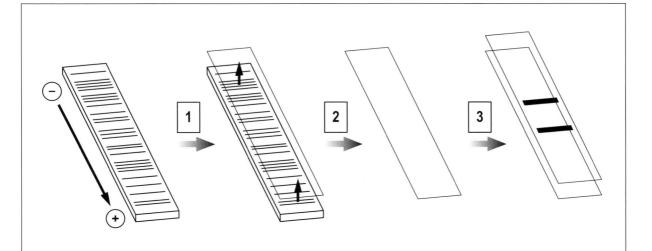

Fig. A3.4 Southern blotting. Step 1: Electrophoresis. Step 2: DNA transfer and fixation. Step 3: Hybridization and autoradiography. Dark bands indicate where probe has bound to homologous sequences.

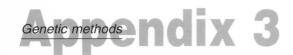

Polymerase chain reaction

By far the most significant advance in genetics in the last few years has been the development of the **polymerase chain reaction** (PCR). This technique allows specific sequences of DNA to be amplified through many orders of magnitude in a quick, relatively simple enzymatic process involving the synthesis of new copies of the chosen sequence (Fig. A3.5). Briefly, the section of genetic material to be amplified is selected from those sections of the genome whose sequence is known, and short synthetic pieces of DNA (**oligonucleotides**) are synthesized chemically to match parts of this region. These molecules (primers) define the section of the genome that will be copied by use of a DNA polymerizing enzyme. The enzyme adds nucleotides to each primer, which has recognized and bound to its complementary sequence, forming a new chain of DNA. Because each strand of the target molecule is copied, the amount of material doubles. The process may be repeated many times, each cycle doubling the material resulting from the previous one. This means that the number of copies of the sequence being amplified increases at an exponential rate. The capacity to amplify quickly and specifically a chosen sequence from a small sample makes this a very powerful technique. PCR can be used to clone genes, probe their structure, mutate them and quantify their expression. This technique is now used routinely in diagnostics, forensics and almost every branch of medical and biological research.

Measuring gene expression

Molecular biologists frequently want to determine where a particular gene is expressed. In addition, the ability to determine when a gene is expressed (and in what amount) allows us to draw conclusions about the involvement of that gene in a particular process, be it developmental, homeostatic or pathogenic. Routinely, researchers use **Northern blotting** (a type of Southern blotting for RNA) to assess gene expression but, recently, newer techniques such as **reverse transcriptase PCR** (RT-PCR) and in situ **hybridization** have added greater sensitivity and refinement.

Northern blotting

Northern blotting is performed on either isolated total RNA or purified mRNA. As with Southern blotting, molecules are separated on the basis of size by electrophoresis and transferred to a membrane by capillary action. The tendency of RNA molecules to form secondary structures (which are likely to affect mobility) requires gels to be run under denaturing conditions. This is a robust technique but it does suffer from limited sensitivity and requires the use of large amounts of tissue to provide sufficient mRNA. Northern blotting allows comparisons of gene expression but can only localize expression to a single tissue or broad region.

Quantitative PCR

PCR is much more sensitive than the other available techniques. Reverse transcriptase is used to produce a cDNA copy of the mRNA to act as a template for the reaction (Fig. A3.6). cDNA synthesis is primed by either oligo-dT (specific for the poly-A tails of mRNA molecules) or the downstream (3′) PCR primer. Theoretically RT-PCR is capable of detecting a single target molecule, but considerable care must be taken to guard against the possibility of false positives resulting from contamination of a sample with previously amplified material. Detecting expression is relatively straightforward but accurate quantification is more difficult. Care must be taken to control for variations in efficiency at all stages: sample preparation, reverse transcription and amplification.

In situ hybridization

Because each tissue is made up of different types of cell, each expressing a slightly different set of genes, it is often important to be able to localize gene expression to specific cell types within a tissue. Sections of fixed or frozen tissue are mounted on microscope slides and subjected to limited proteolysis to allow probe to enter the cells. Probes must be small (to allow them access to the cell) and be labelled to high specific activity – often cocktails of oligonucleotides are used. Non-radioactive labelling methods such as digoxigenin are increasingly favoured for their superior resolution. Tissue can be counterstained with histological stains to aid identification of individual cells.

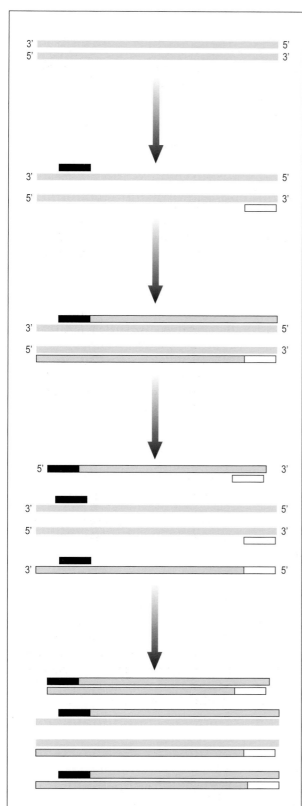

Fig. A3.5 The polymerase chain reaction. Step 1: Denaturation of template and annealing of upstream (filled bar) and downstream (open bar) primers. Step 2: Extension of primers by DNA polymerase to produce new strands of DNA. Step 3: Denaturation and annealing of primers (to both the original template and the newly synthesized strands). Step 4: Extension of primers by DNA polymerase to produce new strands of DNA.

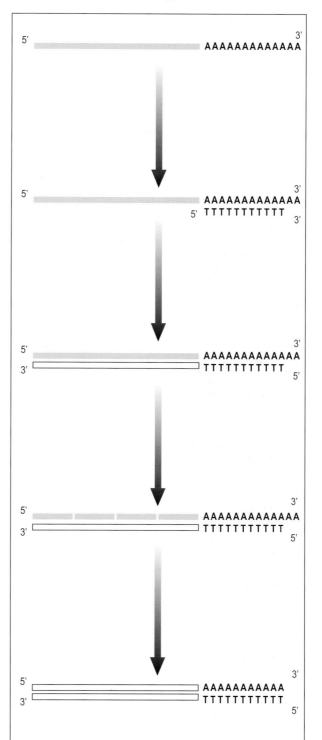

Fig. A3.6 Synthesis of cDNA by reverse transcription. (1) Annealing of oligo-dT primer to poly-A tail of mRNA transcript. (2) Synthesis of first strand by reverse transcriptase (RNA-dependent DNA polymerase) to produce a DNA:RNA hybrid. (3) Nicking of RNA strand of DNA:RNA hybrid by RNase H. (4) Synthesis of second strand by DNA polymerase I, producing a double-stranded cDNA molecule. The range and abundance of cDNA molecules synthesized from an RNA sample is representative of the levels of gene expression in the source tissue. Second strand synthesis is unnecessary if the cDNA is to be used as a template for PCR. Note: Steps 3 and 4 occur simultaneously, but are shown separately here for clarity.

Appendix 3

Linkage

Many diseases have a genetic component. For some such as cystic fibrosis, a defect in a single gene (CFTR) is enough to cause the disease. Other diseases such as hypertension or diabetes may be more complicated, with many genes having the potential to contribute to the condition without any one, on its own, being sufficient to cause it. In these cases there is a need for other factors (genetic or environmental) to be present as well. The genetic defects responsible for many single gene disorders have now been identified by linkage analysis (Fig. A3.7). This involves analysing the DNA of families in whom the disease is prevalent and trying to identify which part of their genetic material an individual has inherited from each parent and determining whether a particular allele is found only in those who develop the disease. In order to carry out a linkage study it is necessary to have a means of distinguishing the different alleles of a gene. There are two ways in which this is achieved: either by using **restriction fragment length polymorphisms** (RFLPs) or **microsatellites**.

RFLP analysis

Southern blots probed with a gene probe will show a characteristic pattern of bands depending on the frequency and location of recognition sites for the restriction endonuclease that is used. If there are no sites within the region recognized by the probe then a single band will be observed. If there is a single site, two bands will be seen, and so on. If one compares the DNA of two individuals, different patterns are sometimes observed, which result from differences (or mutations) in the sequence of the gene (Fig. A3.8). These can result from small changes such as the alteration of a single base, which either deletes an old or creates a new recognition sequence for the enzyme. This is called **point mutation**. Alternatively, changes in pattern may reflect larger alterations in gene structure such as the insertion or deletion of a section of DNA. Sometimes these changes alter the expression or function of the gene, but often they have no effect (i.e. they are 'silent'). Whatever their effect, RFLPs are often very useful for distinguishing between different alleles of a particular gene and can be used to map the structure of the genome of an organism.

Microsatellites

These are short, repetitive, highly polymorphic sequences that occur frequently throughout mammalian genomes. The repeating unit may be just a simple dinucleotide (CACACACACA, etc.) or a more complex sequence. The polymorphic nature of these sequences, which do not appear to have any function, makes them ideal for use as markers for genetic analysis. Often the number of repeat units varies between individuals and their DNA may be distinguished by comparing the size of their microsatellites by PCR or Southern blotting. The highly polymorphic nature of microsatellites is the basis for the technique of DNA fingerprinting, which has revolutionized forensic science. In contrast to RFLPs, microsatellite markers are often not associated with a particular gene, instead identifying just an anonymous region of chromosome. Markers such as these are also being used to map entire genomes (including the human genome) and to locate genes responsible for a wide variety of diseases such as schizophrenia, diabetes and hypertension.

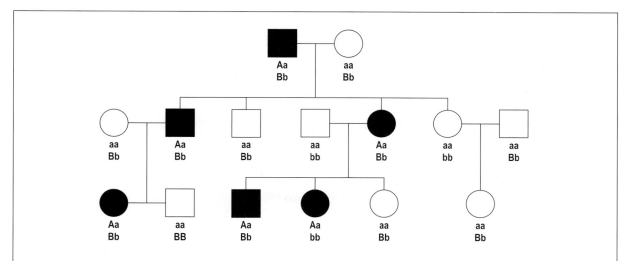

Fig. A3.7 A simple family pedigree, showing the inheritance of two genes, each with two alleles (A or a, and B or b). Affected individuals are indicated as filled shapes. The trait is dominantly inherited and shows linkage to allele A.

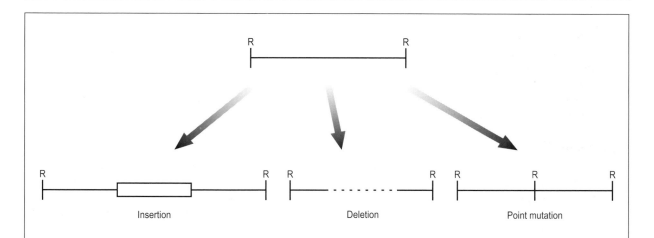

Fig. A3.8 Restriction fragment length polymorphism. Three mechanisms by which the restriction pattern for a specific restriction endonuclease (R) may change: insertion of DNA between the restriction sites, deletion of DNA or point mutation resulting in the creation (or deletion) of a site for enzyme R.

Voltage clamp

Various factors can complicate the measurement of different channel activities in membranes:

- Membrane potential can influence the opening and closing of many types of ion channels.
- Membrane potential influences the driving force on different ions. Thus, where membrane potential is changing rapidly, as in an action potential, the interpretation of electrical recordings is highly complex.
- Current carried by ions through open channels can itself change the membrane potential.

Voltage clamp permits control of the membrane potential and overcomes the normally complex interdependence of membrane potential and channel activity. Voltage clamp is achieved using a feedback amplifier, which resists any change in membrane potential (Fig. A4.1). When current begins to flow through an open channel, the amplifier imposes a current just big enough to resist the channel current. This imposed current can be recorded and gives a measure of the channel activity. By clamping the membrane, potential alterations in channel activity caused by changes in membrane potential are eliminated. This allows the activity of ligand-gated channels to be distinguished from voltage-activated channel activities in the same membrane. Moreover, by stepping the membrane potential to a new value, the response of voltage-sensitive channels to voltage changes can be studied.

Patch clamp

Patch clamp is a method for recording currents from a small patch of membrane and can allow recordings of single channel activity. The patch of membrane is isolated by pressing a glass micropipette (tip diameter < 1 μm) against the cell. The micropipette tips are polished to prevent penetration of the cell and the membrane forms an electrical seal with the pipette, thus isolating a patch of membrane. Four modes of recording are then possible (Fig. A4.2):

1. cell-attached or on-cell recording. In this configuration permeabilization of the patch with nystatin can allow ionic continuity between the cell and patch electrode without dialysis into the micropipette of cellular proteins. This can be important when measuring channel activities that are dependent on intracellular constituents, e.g. phosphorylation by kinases
2. inside-out patch (by pulling off the patch of membrane from the cell)
3. whole-cell recording (by sucking out the patch of membrane through the pipette), and
4. outside-out patch (by pulling off the micropipette from the whole-cell configuration).

Understanding electrophysiological records

By convention, inward currents are shown as a downward deflection on a current versus time plot and outward currents as an upward deflection (Fig. A4.3). This convention is maintained for patch clamp records, even though the patch may be inside-out, etc.

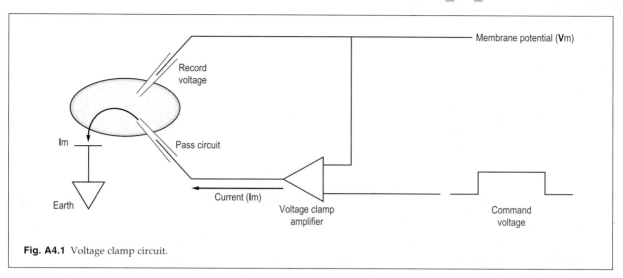

Fig. A4.1 Voltage clamp circuit.

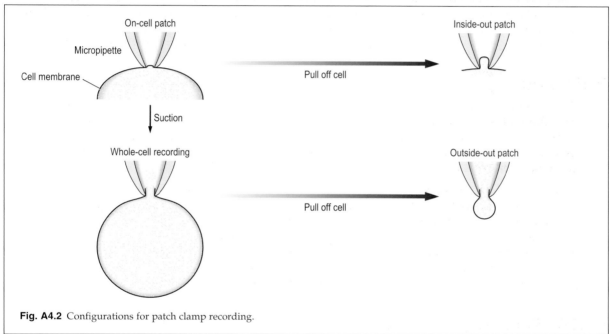

Fig. A4.2 Configurations for patch clamp recording.

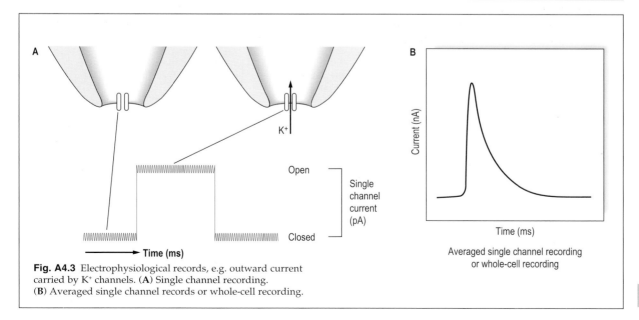

Fig. A4.3 Electrophysiological records, e.g. outward current carried by K⁺ channels. (**A**) Single channel recording. (**B**) Averaged single channel records or whole-cell recording.

Index